# CHIROPRACTIC
## *A Patient's Guide*

An introduction to chiropractic, a manipulative therapy
based on the work of Dr Daniel David Palmer in the
nineteenth century. The therapy is widely recognized and is
continuing to flourish.

# CHIROPRACTIC
## A Patient's Guide

*by*

Dr Michael B. Howitt Wilson
MB, BS, MRCS, LRCP, DObstRCOG, DC

THORSONS PUBLISHING GROUP
Wellingborough, Northamptonshire

———————— • ————————

Rochester, Vermont

First Published 1987

© MICHAEL B. HOWITT WILSON 1987

British Library Cataloguing in Publication Data

Wilson, Michael B. Howitt
Chiropractic: a patient's guide. —
(A Patient's guide)
1. Chiropractic — Great Britain
I. Title II. Series
615.5'34'0941          RZ225.G7

ISBN 0-7225-1201-5

Printed and bound in Great Britain

# Contents

# Acknowledgements

Damian Wilson and Gel Simon have illustrated this book. I am exceedingly grateful to them for contributing to it what I could not.

I owe a great personal debt to the Anglo-European College of Chiropractic for having taught me the science and art of chiropractic, and to the British Chiropractic Association for having allowed a physician to join their ranks.

# Introduction

As medical science has advanced, people have become less concerned with just staying alive, and more with the quality of their lives. They have become less tolerant of minor ailments, and expect to feel well. In an attempt to treat every complaint, doctors have prescribed more medicines and used more sophisticated methods of investigation. At the same time they have had less direct contact with their patients, much of the investigation having been taken over by machines and microprocessors.

A group of disorders which appears to be on the increase, in an age of sedentary occupations and motor cars, is back pain and musculoskeletal disorders. Spinal manipulation is an art which is as old as history, yet it has acquired an ever greater relevance at a time when, although fatal diseases are less threatening, back pain has become one of the greatest causes of absenteeism from work. At the same time it involves direct contact between doctor and patient, uses no drugs, and has an exceptional record of safety.

Of all spinal manipulators, the largest group is the chiropractors, of whom there are over 40,000 worldwide. They grew through the insight of an itinerant healer, Daniel David Palmer, and the enthusiasm of his son B. J. Palmer, an indefatigable eccentric. At the turn of the last century, they sought to supplant medicine thinking they had found the cause of all disease. Instead, they discovered a gap in medicine. A group of common ailments existed which was not appropriately treated either by medicine or by surgery. These ailments required the manual skills of the chiropractor.

In England, chiropractors are becoming increasingly recognized as a highly trained professional body of experts in spinal manipulative therapy. They look forward to the day when they will be fully accepted and integrated into the country's health care system.

It is hoped that this book will help to acquaint the reader with chiropractic. It will demonstrate that, whilst the results of chiropractic treatment can be truly spectacular, it is not magic, but is based on just as sound principles as other therapies which are considered orthodox. In time therefore it must become a part of orthodoxy.

Michael B. Howitt Wilson

## Chapter 1

# What is Chiropractic?

Although the first chiropractic treatment took place in Davenport, Iowa, in 1895, and chiropractic has enjoyed a phenomenal success in North America, it has, until very recently, remained relatively little known in Great Britain. Many people confuse the chiropractor with the chiropodist, and even those who have seen a chiropractor are wont to describe him as their 'back man' or their 'bone man'. Back man he is. About 50 per cent of his patients come to him because of back pain. Bone man he is not. His province is not diseases of bone, but disturbances of the moveable parts adjoining them.

There are about 250 chiropractors in Britain at present. The number is increasing, however, since the first European college (the Anglo-European College of Chiropractic) was founded in 1965, in Bournemouth. This moved to larger premises, formerly Boscombe Convent, in 1981.

Chiropractors are practitioners of a branch of medicine which is concerned with the correction of disordered joint mechanics, especially in the vertebral column. Chiropractic is a branch of medicine, in that it aims to prevent, cure or alleviate disease, but it has still to find its place alongside orthodox medical specialities. Use of the hands in manual operations is by tradition the prerogative of the surgeon. The old word chirurgeon has the same origin as the word chiropractor (Greek: cheir — hand). Surgery, however, is usually associated with the use of the knife. Chiropractors could be said to practise bloodless surgery.

It is a common fallacy to suppose that a chiropractor replaces displaced bones. How often are patients heard to say: 'There was a bone out in my neck, and he put it back'. You have only to think how impossible it is to remain still for any length of time, to realize that bones are in continuous motion at the joints. To say that a bone is displaced can only mean that it has moved outside the normal range for that joint. That would be described as 'dislocation' and would be outside the range of the chiropractor's practice. Chiropractors often use the word 'subluxation'. This term requires a word of explanation, particularly as it is used in a different sense by medical practitioners. To the medical doctor or surgeon, the word suggests a small degree of dislocation. To the chiropractor, it means that the bone appears to be out of alignment relative to the one below, either when inspected visually, or on feeling it, or on the X-ray film. It has come to mean the kind of abnormality which the chiropractor looks for and treats, even when there is no misalignment. It is in fact an abnormality of movement. A bone can be out of alignment because it is not moving in harmony with its neighbours. It can also happen because there is an abnormal muscle pull on that bone, or because movement is not taking place at all, or is taking place in an abnormal manner at an adjacent joint. It is this type of dysfunction of muscles and joints which responds to chiropractic.

The bones of the spine are called vertebrae. Each vertebra is joined to those above and below, not by simple joints, like those of the fingers, but by a complex system called, after a description by the German researcher Herbert Junghanns, the 'intervertebral motor unit'. The parts of this motor unit which permit movement between pairs of vertebrae are three joints. The joint between the bodies (the solid cylindrical parts) of the vertebrae consists mainly of the 'disc'. This is a soft shock-absorber which with the vertebral bodies forms a continuous flexible column in front of the spinal cord. Behind the cord are two projections, called apophyses, which glide over similar structures projecting upwards from the vertebra below. The disc is made of cartilage (gristle). The posterior joints are lined

**Vertebrae**

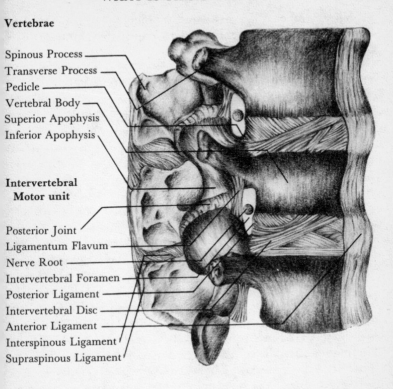

Spinous Process
Transverse Process
Pedicle
Vertebral Body
Superior Apophysis
Inferior Apophysis

**Intervertebral
Motor unit**

Posterior Joint
Ligamentum Flavum
Nerve Root
Intervertebral Foramen
Posterior Ligament
Intervertebral Disc
Anterior Ligament
Interspinous Ligament
Supraspinous Ligament

Figure 1   Vertebrae and Intervertebral Motor Unit (Lateral View)

with cartilage, which in turn is lined with a membrane secreting a lubricating fluid called synovia. The amount of movement possible in each direction at a particular motor unit is controlled by the shape and orientation of the posterior joints (facets), as well as by the disc.

The disorder referred to above as a subluxation is in fact a functional derangement of the motor unit. It may be excessive mobility (a hypermobile subluxation), or restricted mobility (a hypomobile subluxation, or fixation). Such fixations may be partial (that is, on one side only) or total, in which the segment is completely blocked. It is obviously easier to correct loss of mobility, rather than excessive mobility, by manipulation. Thus it is more often the fixations which the chiropractor is looking to treat.

## Chiropractic Theories

The posterior half of a vertebra is called the vertebral arch. On it are located the posterior joints. The parts of the arch which join the articular processes or apophyses (forming the posterior joints) to the vertebral bodies on each side of the vertebral foramen (through which the spinal cord passes) are called the pedicles. Bounded by a pedicle above and another below is an oval channel, the intervertebral foramen, through which passes, among other things, one of the paired segmental nerves which send messages to and from the spinal cord. The front wall of the foramen is part of each of two vertebral bodies and the disc between them. The back wall is the posterior joint between those vertebrae.

Daniel David Palmer, the founder of chiropractic, spoke of subluxated vertebrae impinging on nerves. For him, energy from the brain was transmitted via the spinal cord and spinal nerves to every organ of the body as nerve force. Vertebrae impinging upon the spinal nerves caused either too much or too little nerve force to flow. The place where a nerve is likely to be impinged upon was of course in the intervertebral foramen through which it left the spine. This impingement could cause irritation and excitation (increased nerve force), or it could, by pressure, impede the flow of energy (decreased nerve force).

A number of D. D. Palmer's followers simplified his theory and talked only in terms of 'pinched nerves' causing insufficient nerve energy to reach the various organs of the body, thereby interfering with their function. It was also thought that abnormal function in a particular organ would always be associated with subluxations at specific levels of the spine. This was a grossly oversimplified theory of the cause of disease. Nevertheless, nerve roots do sometimes get compressed as they emerge from the foramina. Pain and symptoms such as 'pins and needles' in the area of the skin supplied by a particular

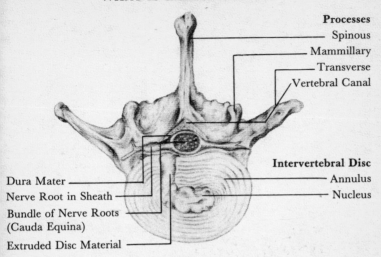

Processes
Spinous
Mammillary
Transverse
Vertebral Canal

Intervertebral Disc
Annulus
Nucleus

Dura Mater
Nerve Root in Sheath
Bundle of Nerve Roots
(Cauda Equina)
Extruded Disc Material

Figure 2    Lumbar Intervertebral Disc Prolapse

nerve suggest that it is being irritated. Numbness and paralysis of muscles are produced by more severe compression. Professor Chung Ha Suh and his fellow researchers at the Department of Mechanical Engineering of the University of Colorado in Boulder, Colorado, have demonstrated in animals that nerves are very much more sensitive to compression at their roots than further down the nerve trunks. It is interesting to note that sciatica was thought to be due to compression of the trunk of the sciatic nerve by the muscles in the buttock, until two surgeons from Boston, W. J. Mixter and J. S. Barr, described the prolapsed disc, in a paper in the *New England Journal of Medicine* in 1934. This paper has become a classic. The two surgeons showed that the nerve was compressed at the level of its roots by protrusion of disc material, and that removal of the extruded disc substance, at operation, relieved the sciatic symptoms. It has also been shown that pressure on nerve roots can interfere with the blood supply to the nerve, as well as with the transport or nutrient substances which normally travel along the nerve fibre itself.

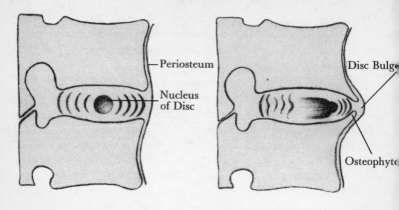

Figure 3    Formation of Osteophytes

Another suggestion was that spinal subluxations could cause pressure on or irritation of the spinal cord itself in the spinal canal. Now we know that degenerative disease of the spine, (spondylosis) can cause spinal cord irritation. As a disc degenerates, it becomes squeezed out between adjacent vertebrae. Disc protrusions carry with them the membrane which is on the surface of all bones including vertebrae, the periosteum. The periosteum's function is to form new bone. Spicules of bone, called osteophytes, or even fringes of bone all round the edges of the vertebrae are thus formed. Such excrescences of bone and disc material can not only narrow intervertebral foramina, but can also encroach on the vertebral foramen, through which the spinal cord passes, narrowing it. Also well documented is pressure on the cord from displacement of the upper two vertbrae in the neck (the atlas and axis) caused by loosening of the ligaments holding them. This can happen because of infection or diseases such as rheumatoid arthritis, which attack the ligaments (the holding bands which normally prevent joints from moving too far). Asymmetrical contraction of the small muscles attached to the atlas, can hold it in a distorted position or produce excessive excursion of the atlas. This may also cause spinal cord symptoms. Severe compression of the cord would lead to paralysis of all four limbs or even to death. Minor degrees of cord compression, however, cause headache, loss of balance and tingling in the hands and feet.

Passing through the bones of the neck via a hole (the foramen transversarium) which exists on either side of the vertebral foramen are a pair of arteries called the vertebral arteries. These can be pressed on or irritated by abnormal movements or positions of the neck vertebrae. Each artery normally passes through the upper six vertebrae and winds round the back of the joints between the atlas and the base of the skull. Compression of these arteries may produce headache, vertigo or dizziness, nausea and 'drop attacks' in which the legs become suddenly, temporarily paralysed, and the person falls to the ground.

Perhaps the most common effect of abnormal function of the motor unit is pain. Pain can arise from pressure on sensitive structures such as the sheath of dura mater covering the spinal cord and the nerve roots arising from it. It can also be caused by abnormal tension on ligaments and on the fibrous capsules of the posterior spinal joints as well as by spasm of muscles, which contract in response to injury or threatened injury to joints. Such pain can be felt locally, at the site of irritation, or it can be referred. Referred pain is pain felt at a distance from its cause. It occurs because a number of structures are supplied by nerves from the same segment of the spinal cord, which also supplies an area of skin. Thus pain from the upper part of the lumbar spine is often felt in the groin, and pain from the lower lumbar spine on the top of the foot. Pain felt anywhere in the body could be arising from the spine and this site of origin is often forgotten. That is why pain originating in the spinal column frequently mimics other conditions.

Probably the most important structures affected by disturbed function in the spine are the nerves of position sense (proprioception). These tell our central nervous system what position our joints are in, and what state of contraction each muscle is in. Such nerve endings are present in all joints and in their muscles and ligaments, and are affected by alterations in stretch or pressure. We should be unable to stand up if alterations in posture in one part of the body were not automatically compensated by postural changes elsewhere. Thus increased tone in the muscles of one side of the lumbar spine produces increased tone in the muscles of the opposite side of the neck. Change of tone in the neck muscles will also affect the lumbar region. It is not surprising, therefore, to find that there is never just one fixation in a person's spine, but always a series of them. A mechanical disturbance in one joint causes a chain reaction. It is quite possible that a pain in the neck may be caused by a disturbance of the mechanics of the pelvis. Stimulation of the nerve endings monitoring tension (often called mechanoreceptors) causes muscle spasm, or increased muscle tone, not only locally and in other parts of the spine, but also in muscle groups at a distance from the spine. This occurs especially in those muscles which have the same segmental nerve supply as the affected joint. The degree of pain felt when pain-sensitive nerve endings are stimulated is also influenced by the input to the central nervous system of impulses from these mechanoreceptors.

It is clear that disturbance of the mechanics of the spine may have various and profound effects on the body as a whole, the most common of which are pain syndromes.

## Adjustment of Spinal Joints

We have seen that the principal target of chiropractic treatment is the subluxation. The subluxation may signify excessive or limited mobility in the intervertebral motor unit, that is in the moving parts between the bones of the spine. In general, excessive mobility in one motor unit is associated with decreased movement (fixation) elsewhere. There is little point in manipulating a segment which is already too mobile. Manipulation is best suited to mobilizing segments which have become fixed — that is, whose mobility is limited. An adjustment is a manipulation used to start a fixed or partially immobilized joint moving again. It is essentially a method of

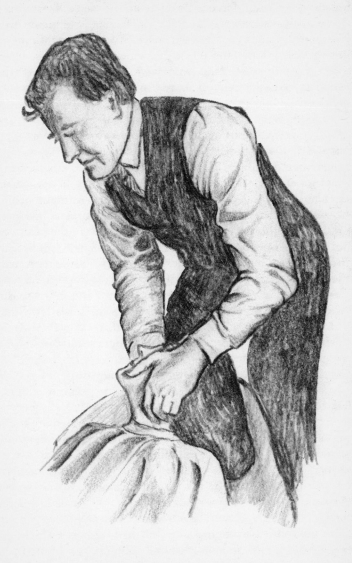

Figure 4    A Cervical Adjustment

applying a sudden force across a joint in such a way as to momentarily separate the joint surfaces. You may have experienced one of your fingers feeling not quite right and not moving freely. Cracking the appropriate knuckle immediately restored it to normal. That is analogous to what a chiropractor does when he adjusts a joint. In the spine, of course, the fixation is likely to be more definite, and to produce greater effects, not only on the fixed joint, but on other structures as well.

I have spoken of an adjustment as restoring movement to a joint which is fixed or jammed. The effects of subluxations on muscle tone has been discussed. The adjustment also has a profound effect on muscle tone. When the muscles closely associated with a joint are in spasm, an adjustment usually causes an immediate reduction in the degree of spasm. Muscles at a distance may also be affected, and indeed other fixations may also be released. This effect occurs through the sudden stimulation of mechanoreceptors. It is as if a circuit were suddenly interrupted, allowing a 'rebalancing' of muscle tone. There is often a more direct effect on a small muscle in spasm. If the ends of that muscle are suddenly pulled apart, so as to exert a rapid stretch on the muscle, then it will react by relaxing. This again is a reflex action operating through the central nervous system.

Apart from reflex effects on muscles, an adjustment forcefully separates joint surfaces. These apparently become adherent after being held immobile. The joint surfaces literally become stuck together, and are physically separated by the manipulation. In longstanding or chronic fixations, ligaments will have become shorter. Such joints may have to be adjusted a number of times over a period to induce movement and persuade liagaments to lengthen. In the same way, joints which have become excessively mobile tend to stabilize once the stress is taken off them by restoring movement to neighbouring joints.

The chiropractor attempts to restore function to the spine and often to peripheral joints as well. He has to proceed bit by bit. Each adjustment has a profound effect. Every action which improves function in one part of the spine improves the function of the whole spine. Doing too much at once can upset things, a second adjustment, or another procedure, sometimes acting in opposition to what has already been achieved. When a spinal joint is adjusted, muscles are released from a state of irritation and spasm, and assume a normal tone. It is only too easy to cause renewed irritation by further manipulation. Once an adjustment has been allowed to develop its full effect, the spine can be re-assessed and further treatment be given.

## Osteopathy and Chiropractic

Whenever manipulative techniques are discussed, the question always arises: 'What is the difference between osteopaths and chiropractors?' It is not easy to give an accurate straight answer, as both treat similar conditions using techniques which are essentially the same. The two schools, which were both founded in the USA, have grown up separately.

Chiropractors in England have studied either at the Anglo-European College of Chiropractic in Bournemouth, or at one of the eighteen North American colleges. They use the letters DC (Doctor of Chiropractic) to show their qualification, and most of them belong to the British Chiropractic Association. Osteopaths are either MRO (Member of the Register of Osteopaths) and are graduates of the British School of Osteopathy or medical practitioners who have taken a thirteen-month part-time course at the London College of Osteopathic Medicine. Alternatively, they may be MBNOA (Member of the British Naturopathic and Osteopathic Association) and have qualified at the British College of Osteopathy and Naturopathy, or MSO (Member of the Society of Osteopaths) which is an offshoot of the BNOA concentrating on manipulative therapy. Naturopathic practitioners make extensive use of dietary advice as an essential part of their therapy and may use acupuncture, herbalism and homoeopathy. In the USA osteopaths have been absorbed into the medical profession. Many have therefore become more medical, and less manipulative, practitioners, and some practise surgery. In England, they are in the same position as chiropractors, having no officially recognized status. There is less diversity among chiropractors, who have retained manipulation as their forte.

Originally, the philosophies of the two disciplines were different. Whereas both believed that the body's natural resources could be mobilized to heal disease, if spinal lesions or subluxations were eliminated by manipulation, the osteopaths believed that this was achieved by improvement in circulation of blood to organs. The chiropractors believed it happened by permitting proper functioning of the nervous system. These differences have now faded into history. Chiropractors are proud of the fact that as chiropractic was discovered in the same year as X-rays, 1895, they make full use of diagnostic radiography. X-rays are used more in chiropractic than in osteopathic diagnosis. There are general differences in techniques used. The chiropractor uses rapid, low-amplitude thrusts directly on to one of the bones adjacent to a joint. The point of contact is on the vertebra to be moved, and speed is of the essence. He may use other techniques, but his adjustments are such that they can be performed with little or no preparation. The osteopath does more soft tissue work (superficial and deep massage), mobilizes the joints by traction or articulation (putting joints through their full range of movement passively) and finally may deliver a more specific thrust, often a long-lever move with the point of contact at a distance from the joint to be moved.

## Structure and Function

It is to Andrew Taylor Still (1828-1912), the founder of osteopathy, that the saying 'structure governs function' is attributed. In fact, it seems to be mainly surgeons who work on this principle. Should an orthopaedic or a neurosurgeon see a narrow spinal canal, with the possibility of pressure on spinal nerves and their blood supply, his instinct is to widen it. Should he see a disc prolapse or bulge, his instinct is to remove it. Sometimes such measures are necessary, but such operations are not always successful. Careful examination of the movement at individual intervertebral motor units after disc surgery will often reveal excessive mobility amounting to instability. This dysfunction may well be responsible for residual symptoms. John Hilton (1804-78), a surgeon of Guy's Hospital, London, wrote a book in 1863 which stressed the importance of rest in the treatment of painful conditions. This book has a great influence on surgical treatment. Indeed, if one rests a painful back, it will usually improve. Commonly, however, some loss of function remains, causing persistence or recurrence of symptoms.

The chiropractor looks for abnormal function. Reduced, excessive or abnormal movements of individual spinal joints leads to disharmony in the working of the spinal column as a whole. His adjustments help to correct the mechanical function of the spine, thereby improving the health of joints, ligaments, muscles and nerves. Disuse of joints and muscles causes atrophy (wasting), thereby altering their structure; so, it would be more accurate to state that function governs structure. Even changes which have occurred in cartilage and bone can improve with restoration of function, although admittedly they are very slow in healing. This applies particularly to cartilage, as it has no blood supply. It is therefore all the more important to prevent deterioration. The chiropractor does this by allowing joints and muscles to be used normally, and by removing abnormal stresses.

## Safety of Manipulation

One of the things which is often said about manipulation in general and about chiropractic in particular, is that it is dangerous. Nothing could be farther from the truth. J. P. Ladermann, a chiropractor from Geneva, reviewing the literature on the subject in 1981, found 135 cases described of accidents associated with spinal manipulation, among which fourteen deaths occurred. The papers referred to were published between 1907 to 1980, a period of seventy-three years. It is difficult to be sure that the effects described in many of these cases were in fact due to the manipulation. On the other hand, there must have been many accidents which did not appear in the literature. If one compares these figures with the number of unfavourable reactions to and deaths from, say, aspirin, they are infinitesimal. In the USA there are 34,000 chiropractors. They alone must perform at least half a million adjustments a day. If accidents were happening frequently, they would be reported every day. The law courts would have been kept very busy with such cases. It is a fact that compared with physicians and surgeons, chiropractors pay very small malpractice insurance premiums.

We can conclude that spinal manipulative therapy in the hands of a qualified chiropractor is one of the safer forms of treatment, and that accidents, though not unknown, are rare and usually not serious. One reason is that the patient is awake, and so his natural defensive reactions are unimpaired. Most chiropractors view with horror the idea of manipulating under general anaesthetic, a procedure frequently carried out in hospital practice. Anaesthesia not only makes the procedure more hazardous by stopping the patient from resisting painful movements, but also adds the danger of the anaesthetic, which is itself not without risks.

Treatment by a chiropractor usually involves manipulation. This is his area of expertise. Most patients will need a number of adjustments, and the benefit may not be immediately obvious. Often they ask themselves after a few sessions: 'Is it doing any good?' They sometimes worry that the chiropractor may 'overmanipulate'. This attitude is understandable, but is usually based on a misconception of what a chiropractor is doing.

It is possible to overmanipulate, but this usually involves manipulating a joint which should not have been touched in the first place. Thus to manipulate a joint which is already moving too much (a hypermobile joint) can make it worse. On the other hand, not to manipulate a joint which is immobile may be permitting degenerative changes to occur when they could have been avoided or minimized. As long as the chiropractor restricts his activities to joints which are hypomobile (fixations), he cannot overmanipulate. Once mobility is restored, he will no longer need to manipulate that joint. As we have already seen, fixations do not usually occur singly. Disturbed mechanics in one part of the spine will invariably affect other parts. Even fixations of joints apart from the vertebral column, such as those of the feet, upset the spine. It is therefore unusual for one adjustment to completely correct a problem. Each adjustment will improve the function of the joint adjusted, and of the spine as a whole, but the healing processes of the body must be allowed to operate between treatments. Thus a number of adjustments are necessary at intervals of a few days. Chronic or longstanding fixations, where there has been loss of function for a prolonged period, are associated with degenerative changes in bone, cartilage, ligaments and muscles. It can sometimes be necessary to adjust these on a number of occasions for function to be restored.

In a survey carried out by Alan Breen, a chiropractor from Salisbury, between 1973 and 1974, the average number of adjustments (or rather, treatment sessions) to optimum benefit was seven. Optimum benefit was attained before the eleventh visit in 80 per cent of cases. Nearly 20 per cent of patients therefore required more than eleven treatment sessions to attain optimum benefit. This cannot be said to be overmanipulation. The wonderful thing about chiropractic is that, slowly but surely, painful conditions which have been troublesome for many years gradually improve. 'Miracle cures' in which acute pain disappears with one adjustment, are of course observed by every chiropractor, but only once in a while.

Another area in which chiropractors may be misunderstood is their attitude to prevention. It is a common experience for chiropractors to find mechanical disturbances in the spines of patients who are not complaining. Some will prudently leave them alone. Many, however, consider that these silent subluxations are likely to cause trouble in the future, and are inclined to adjust them even though symptomless. This is a form of preventive therapy. It is often suggested that all patients should attend for a check-up about every six months. After all, we do the same for our teeth.

## Definition

What, then, is chiropractic? The definition given by the European Chiropractors' Union in 1968 states:

> Chiropractic is a discipline of the scientific healing arts concerned with pathogenesis, diagnosis, therapeutics and prophylaxis of functional disturbances, pain syndromes and the neurophysiological effects related to static and dynamic disorders of the locomotor system, particularly of the spine and pelvis.

The British Chiropractic Association's definition may be simpler to understand:

> Chiropractic is that independent branch of medicine which specializes in mechanical disorders of the joints, particularly those of the spine, and their effects on the nervous system. Diagnostic methods include X-ray, and treatment is mainly by specific manipulation without the use of drugs or surgery.

## Chapter 2

# History of Chiropractic

### D.D. Palmer: The Discoverer

Daniel David Palmer was born near Toronto, Canada, on 7th March 1845. At the age of 20, he travelled to the United States and became a schoolmaster in Muscatine County, Iowa. In 1871, he bought some land near New Boston where he grew raspberries and kept bees. In 1881, he sold up and moved to What Cheer, Iowa, where his two brothers lived, and where he ran a grocery business and also sold goldfish. D.D., as he became known universally, was an avid reader of the Bible and books on spiritualism. He must have become aware of a gift in the healing sphere as he became interested in the activities of a magnetic healer Paul Caster, and his son J. S. Caster. He studied magnetic healing, which consisted in laying on of hands, much as healers do today, and began to practise it in Burlington, Iowa in 1886, soon moving to Davenport where he built up a thriving practice. During this transition from teacher, through beekeeper, grocer and fish salesman to healer, he was supported by four wives in succession and had one stepson, two daughters and a son by his second wife, Louvenia, who died in 1884.

D.D. seems to have had an insatiable desire to find *the* cause of disease, that is, one cause for all sickness. He also developed an interest in the asssociation between the vertebrae and disease, having been informed by a Dr Jim Atkinson of Davenport, Iowa, that the replacing of displaced vertebrae had been known and practised by the ancient Egyptians for at least 3000 years.

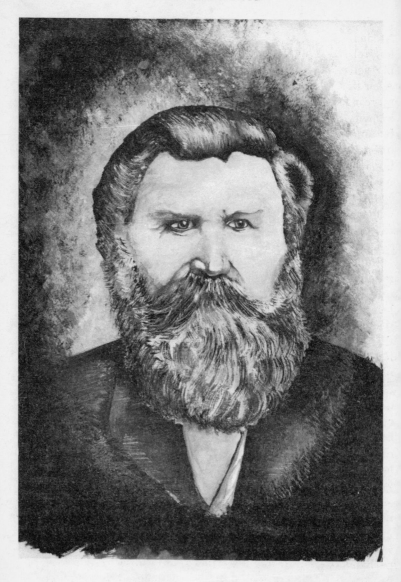

Figure 5    Daniel David Palmer (1844-1913)

We know from his writings that Hippocrates, the Father of Medicine (460-377 BC), used both traction and manipulation for relief of ailments. Galen (AD129-199), also a Greek physician, revived physical treatments of the vertebral column. After this, little is heard of manipulative treatments until much more recent times when we hear of the bonesetters. The best known of these is Mrs Sarah Mapp of Epsom, in England, who became famous in the early eighteenth century. She was unusual, not only in achieving cures which seemed miraculous, but in attracting upper-class clients and making a substantial income. Later in 1867, James Paget (1814–1899), the great Victorian surgeon and teacher of St. Bartholomew's Hospital, was to stress the absence of the manipulative art in medical teaching by lecturing to his students on: 'The Cases that Bone-Setters Cure'.

Palmer claimed, not to have discovered or invented vertebral manipulation, but to have re-discovered it, and to be the first to use the spinous and transverse processes of the vertebrae as levers, to rack the bones of the spine back into place. How did this come about? Harvey Lillard, a janitor in the block where Palmer had his office, had been deaf for seventeen years, so that in D.D. Palmer's words 'he could could not hear the racket of a wagon on the street or the ticking of a watch'. On 18th September 1895, Palmer enquired about the cause of his deafness, and was told that he was exerting himself in a cramped, stooped position, when he felt something give in his back, and immediately became deaf. An examination showed a displaced vertebra, and Palmer managed to persuade Lillard to let him replace it. D.D. Palmer says 'I replaced the 4th dorsal vertebra by one move, which restored his hearing fully'. Shortly afterwards, he found a similarly displaced vertebra in a case of heart trouble. Again he adjusted it with immediate relief.

So D.D. Palmer reasoned that if two such dissimilar diseases were caused by displaced vertebrae impinging on nerves, perhaps other diseases had the same cause. He began to propound his theory that all disease was caused by too much or too little nerve tension, the abnormal state being produced by impingement of vertebrae on the spinal nerves. He thought of nerves as analogous to the strings of musical instruments being impinged upon by the bridge, which affected the rate of vibration thereof. The word 'tone' applied not just to muscles, but also to nerves. Too much or too little tone was the cause of disease.

D.D. started his school, the Palmer Institute and Chiropractic Infirmary, on the fourth floor of the Putnam Building, in Brady Street, Davenport, Iowa. The Reverend Samual H. Weed, a Presbyterian minister, whose wife and daughter had adjustments in 1896, and who himself came for treatment from D.D. was asked to suggest a name for the science and art which he was developing. As spinal manipulation had Greek origins, and D.D. wished it to suggest doing by hand, the Reverend Weed produced the name Chiropractic.

D.D. taught the science, art and philosophy of chiropractic in Davenport from 1896 to 1902. He taught only one or two students at a time. Fifteen had graduated by 1902, in which year four students graduated, one of whom was his son, B. J. (Like his father he was always known by his initials.) D.D. did not run the school on a sound business basis and by 1902 it was in considerable debt. D.D. left his son in control of the school and once again took to the road. His fourth wife died in 1905, and he married his fifth wife in 1906. He practised and taught chiropractic in the Indian Territory, California, Oregon and Canada. He collected notes over the years and in Portland, Oregon, in 1910, he published them as a book called *The Chiropractor's Adjustor*. In it, he castigated not only allopathic medicine, denouncing drugs and vaccination, but also all those who deviated from the pure, unadulterated chiropractic in which he believed: the removal of the cause of disease by adjusting vertebrae. He rebuked those who attempted to re-christen chiropractic and raise it as their own. These included Willard Carver, who founded a rival school, Dr A.P. Davis, one of his first students, who was also a physician and an osteopath, and his own son, B. J.

D.D. returned to Davenport in 1913 to stake his claim as the discoverer and developer of chiropractic. In spite of the fact that he had left the development of the Palmer school to his son, he insisted that he should have the place of honour in the homecoming parade. He tried to walk in front of the parade, waving an American flag. B. J., who was at the wheel of a car, remonstrated with him, and apparently ran into him. D.D. died in Los Angeles three months later, in fact of typhoid. A charge of patricide against his son was not substantiated, but the mud stuck, and it took a long time for the rumours to die down.

If it had not been for his son and the expansion of the school in Davenport, chiropractic would probably have remained the tool of a few privileged individuals for some time. D.D. was not for spreading it about, and would rather have kept it a family affair, certainly until such time as he had worked out the scientific basis. He was pleased to see his teaching influencing others, but equally irritated by seeing it distorted, simplified and diluted. When he saw the growth of the school he had founded he wished to re-instate himself as the Fountainhead. D.D. was a poor businessman, however, and B. J.'s advisors saw that he was not allowed to take over. He died an embittered man, jealous of the success of others with his discovery, and upset that he had lost control of it.

## B. J. Palmer: The Developer

Bartlett Joshua Palmer was born in 1881. He was therefore only 14 years of age when his father performed that first chiropractic adjustment which restored the hearing of Harvey Lillard. Yet he helped his father in the school, and took it over, complete with debts, in 1902, when he was but 21 years of age. B. J. was for expanding and publicizing the new field. In 1904, he bought a large new property in Brady Street and in 1905, the new Palmer School of Chiropractic was incorporated. In 1912, he expanded the school, acquiring adjacent property and erecting new school and administration buildings.

B. J. had a remarkable power of organization. Unlike his

father, he set out to proclaim chiropractic to the world at large. To this end he had a printing press and a radio station in the college. He expanded the osteological museum, which his father had started, to make it the largest collection of human spines in the world — over 10,000 specimens. He had one of the first X-ray laboratories, and his research clinic became one of the finest and best-equipped anywhere. He developed the neurocalometer, an instrument for measuring temperature differences on either side of the spinal column, and then his electroencephaloneuromentimpograph, the forerunner of today's electroencephalograph (EEG) used for recording brain waves.

It is interesting to trace the changes that occurred in B. J. Palmer's teaching over the years. The greatest mistake of the Palmers, as indeed of many in the healing professions, was to expect to find one cause of disease. Nearly all disease can be said to have more than one cause, and certainly different diseases have different causes. Nevertheless, though very different in style and temperament, both the Palmers were driven by the ambition of finding and removing *the* cause of disease.

His first, and possibly most important, discovery was the Palmer recoil adjustment. Whereas his father had used a stiff-arm thrust to deliver an adjustment, requiring a fair amount of force, the recoil adjustment was based on speed, so that it did not need strength to perform. Then he developed the Meric system (Greek: meros — part). The body was divided into thirty-one zones corresponding to the paired spinal nerves, and diseases of different organs were attributed to a subluxation in the appropriate spinal region. Thus, the brain, the eyes, the ears, the pharynx, and the thyroid gland were affected by displacement of one of the four upper cervical vertebrae. Deviation of the fifth to seventh cervical vertebrae caused nose, mouth, throat, lung, shoulder and arm disease. Whooping cough would have been caused by a displacement in this region. And so on down the spinal column. The Meric system enabled the chiropractor to look for displacement of specific vertebrae rather than trying to correct all distortions. He therefore

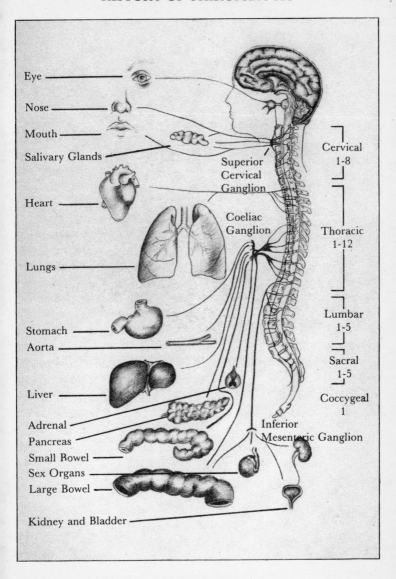

Figure 6   Nerve Supply to Organs via Sympathetic System

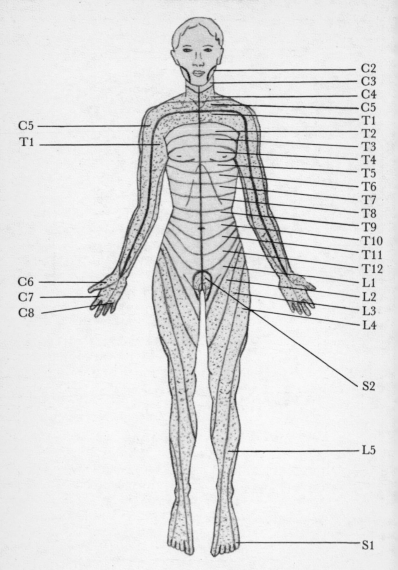

Figure 7    Dermatomes – Segmental Nerve Supply to Skin Zones

concentrated on only a few adjustments. Later, B. J. formulated the theory of majors and minors, in which it was necessary to deal only with certain major subluxations as the minor ones would then go on their own.

B. J. Palmer equipped his own radiographic laboratory only thirteen years after the discovery of X-rays by Wilhelm Roentgen in 1895. By 1909-10, he began teaching the importance of X-rays in visualizing vertebral displacement or subluxation, and lost many friends and followers on this account. Then he became interested in locating 'hot boxes' along the spine. Subluxations produced nerve irritation, which produced heat. In 1923, a member of staff of the Palmer School of Chiropractic, Doss Evins, suggested the possibility of an instrument to locate these hot spots, and B. J. enthusiastically took up with the idea. In August 1924, in a famous address at the annual Palmer School lyceum, 'The Hour Has Struck', B. J. announced the neurocalometer, and asserted that no chiropractor could practise without one. That speech is said to have marked the beginning of the decline of B. J.'s unquestioned leadership of the profession. He met with tremendous opposition from both his friends and his enemies.

In 1930, he announced his latest step in the evolution of the specific spinal adjustment. This was HIO or Hole-in-One Chiropractic. As nerves could be impinged upon by their bony surrounds, so could the spinal cord, and the one place through which all nerves connecting the brain with the body must pass, was the foramen magnum at the base of the skull, and the upper vertebra, the atlas. The atlas was often pulled out of place, causing pressure on the spinal cord, and correction of displacement in this region would remove the cause of all disease. Once again, he alienated many of his supporters and lost many students. Nevertheless, the Palmer School remained the dominant school of chiropractic. Later, B. J. was to return to a more general spinal adjusting.

It is interesting to take a closer look at HIO Chiropractic. It seems the ultimate in naïveté to imagine that a thrust on one particular bone could remove the cause of all disease. Yet B. J.

was able to teach students to perform an adjustment well, since only one technique was required. Only one adjustment was performed per patient visit. Further, upper cervical dysfunction has a greater effect on the body as a whole than dysfunction of any other part of the spine. So, although not the panacea he believed, it was not as ridiculous as some may think.

Until his death in 1961, B. J. stood for pure chiropractic against those whom he saw as practising medicine. It is to him that chiropractic owes its identity. Unlike osteopathy in the USA which became part of the medical profession and almost ceased to exist as a separate entity, chiropractic continued to be independent, both as a profession and in its individual philosophy.

## Mixers and Straights

Willard Carver, an Oklahoma lawyer, founded his own school of chiropractic in Oklahoma City in 1906. He is criticized by D.D. in *The Chiropractors Adjustor* among other things for trying to persuade Palmer that suggestion was a useful adjunct to chiropractic. Carver also believed in supplementing chiropractic with massage, heat therapy, diets and so on. He was a rival of the Palmers for forty years and described himself as 'the Constructor of the Science of Chiropractic'. Right up to the present day there has been disagreement and even hostility between the 'mixers' as portrayed by the Carver school, and the 'straights', followers of the 'pure, straight and unadulterated chiropractic' school of B. J. Palmer. These differences have not yet been reconciled. They remain in the two chiropractic associations of the USA, the American Chiropractic Association (ACA), and the International Chiropractic Association (ICA). There is at present a movement aimed at bringing together the ACA and ICA to form one unified association.

## Prosecutions and Progress

In England a very famous bonesetter, Sir Herbert Barker, came to practise in London in 1906. He had studied bonesetting under his cousin and, in spite of having no medical training nor formal qualifications, he became extremely successful. So successful was he that he was knighted for his services to the nation's health just after the First World War. A Dr Frederick Axham, being greatly impressed with Barker's skills, offered to act as his anaesthetist. For the 'infamous conduct' of assisting an 'unqualified practitioner', Dr Axham's name was struck off the medical register. In England, The General Medical Council could not act against Sir Herbert, who could treat patients under common law, and would only have broken the law had he fraudulently proclaimed himself a registered medical practitioner. Any doctor who willingly assisted him, however, was guilty of infamous conduct, and could be disciplined.

In the United States, things were different. D.D. Palmer was tried, convicted and imprisoned for practising medicine without a certificate from the state board of health, in Scott County, Iowa, in 1906. He served twenty-three days of his 105–day sentence, then was freed following payment of a fine. Hundreds of chiropractors in many states were to face the courts and suffer convictions and jail sentences for practising medicine without a licence, and this continued until the 1960's.

Gradually, chiropractors were accepted by the public, and one by one laws were passed to licence practitioners in all of the United States, and in most countries in which they practise. In England they still practise under common law. In France they still practise illegally. In 1974, the United States Office of Education authorized the Council on Chiropractic Education of the American Chiropractic Association to accredit chiropractic colleges, which thereby received official recognition. In that year also, the last remaining state without a licensing board (Louisiana) started granting licences to chiropractors. In the same year Congress authorized Medicare payments to chiropractors.

In 1975, a conference of the National Institute for Neurological and Communicative Diseases and Stroke, of the United States Public Health Service, discussed 'the scientific basis of spinal manipulative therapy'. Experts in neurology, biomechanics, osteopathy and chiropractic made spinal manipulative therapy a scientifically recognized entity. In 1979, a commission appointed by the Government of New Zealand produced a report of the most thorough enquiry ever made into chiropractic. The commission was not impressed by the objections of the medical profession, said chiropractic could not be dismissed as 'an unscientific cult', and that chiropractors, unlike general practitioners and physiotherapists, were fully trained to carry out spinal diagnosis and therapy at a sophisticated and refined level.

## Chiropractic in Europe

The first chiropractors came to Europe before the First World War. Their numbers gradually grew, and professional associations were formed in several countries. The British Chiropractic Association was established in 1925. At its 6th Annual Conference in 1931, thirty-five members were present plus twenty-one visiting chiropractors from Belgium, Denmark, Sweden and Switzerland. They discussed the formation of an international association to unite European chiropractors, hold annual conferences, further research and compile a register of names and addresses. The European Chiropractic Union was born.

The need for a European college was discussed, but not until 1960 did a group of chiropractors from Britain join with other interested chiropractors from other European countries to form the Anglo-European College of Chiropractic as a charitable organization. A building in Cavendish Road, Bournemouth, was purchased in 1965. The first class was enrolled in September of that year. In 1966, a building opposite was acquired for use as a clinic as well as to provide further classrooms and laboratories. These premises were soon outgrown. In 1981, Boscombe Convent, which had sufficient accommodation for 400 students, was bought and the college moved there.

The Anglo-European College of Chiropractic has helped to swell the ranks of the chiropractic profession in Europe and especially in Britain. The number of chiropractors in Europe is over 1200, and the British Chiropractic Association membership has passed the 200 mark and is growing continuously. Several countries have pre-chiropractic study courses or insist on post-graduate training before full recognition. In France, where chiropractic is considered by law to be a medical act, in order to gain recognition the French National Association of Chiropractors has started its own college, the Institut Francais de Chiropractic, which opened in 1984.

In 1977, in its blue book *Professional Conduct and Discipline: Fitness to Practise*, the General Medical Council stated that it had no desire to restrain the delegation to persons who had been trained to perform specialized functions, of treatment or procedures falling within the proper scope of their skills. It added that a doctor who delegates treatment or other procedures must be satisfied that the person to whom they are delegated is competent to carry them out. Also that the doctor should retain the ultimate responsibility for the management of his patients. This was a far more liberal attitude than that taken at the time of Sir Herbert Barker, and has encouraged greater referral between doctors and chiropractors.

In 1975, the British Chiropractic Association decided to apply for registration under the Professions Supplementary to Medicine Act 1960. Such registration would have given members official status, in the same way as physiotherapists, chiropodists and so on. The application was rejected by the Council for the Professions Supplementary to Medicine without reasons being given. Appeals to the Department of Health and Social Security, to the Privy council and to the Prime Minister were ineffective in altering the position. At present the Anglo-European College of Chiropractic is applying to the Council for National Academic Awards for recognition of its chiropractic training as a degree course. The British Chiropractic Association is co-operating with the Council for Complementary and Alternative Medicine, which also represents other health care disciplines in attempting to gain support from Parliament for legislation.

It will hopefully not be too long before chiropractors in Britain hold a recognized degree, have official status in the health care field, and take their place in provision of treatment under the National Health Service.

## Chapter 3

# Chiropractic Research

**Nerve Root Compression**

In a famous paper written in 1934 in the *New England Journal of Medicine*, as we have already noted in Chapter 1, two Boston surgeons, W. J. Mixter and J. S. Barr, convinced the medical profession that a rupture of the intervertebral disc could produce pressure on nerve roots in the spinal canal and that they could be decompressed surgically. After that, sciatica, which had previously been thought to be due to compression of the great nerve trunk, the sciatic nerve, between muscles deep in the buttock, was understood to be caused by pressure on nerve roots as they emerged from the spinal canal. This confirmed the long-held chiropractic belief that nerve roots could be impinged upon at spinal level. It did, however, change the accent from bony impingement to impingement by cartilaginous disc substance.

Some very impressive research has come from the University of Colorado in recent years. S. K. Sharpless, Ph.D., of the Department of Psychology at that University, working with Professor C. H. Suh showed, by stimulating the dorsal roots and the sciatic nerve trunk in cats whilst applying gentle pressures and measuring the electrical nerve impulse further down the nerve, that much greater pressure on the sciatic nerve was necessary to reduce the impulse than on the roots. Pressures of only 20mm of mercury reduced the action potentials of the dorsal roots by half. (It requires a pressure of 120mm of mercury to occlude the pulse at the wrist). This work is of great interest because it confirms, not only that nerve root

compression is a feasible cause of symptoms, but also that the
impression of many chiropractors that cases labelled as carpal
tunnel syndrome, ulnar tunnel compression, meralgia
paraesthetica and peroneal nerve compression have been
relieved by spinal adjustment. These are conditions in which
nerves are said to be compressed along their course in the limbs.
Obviously one must be careful in assuming that the nerve trunk
is compressed when it could be the nerve root. Spinal
manipulation would then appear to be more logical than
surgical decompression of the nerve in the appropriate tunnel.
There is a hypothesis of a 'double crush' cause of such
symptoms, the nerve being sensitized at root level, and then
being compressed again — for instance, in the medial nerve as
it passes through the carpal tunnel at the wrist, leading to
symptoms in the hand, of pain, weakness, pins and needles and
numbness.

## Spinal Biomechanics

A well-known Swiss chiropractor, F. W. H. Illi of Geneva,
made a detailed study of the sacro-iliac joints and the effects of
distortion of the pelvis on locomotion and the mechanics of the
spine, He was one of the great chiropractic researchers and his
book, *The Vertebral Column, Life-line of the Body*, published in 1951
is a classic of chiropractic literature. Present-day Swiss
chiropractors such as E. Lorez and R. Sandoz have continued
the tradition of inquiry and research and are regular
contributors to the Journal called *Annals of the Swiss Chiropractor's
Association*.

A. E. Homewood, former President of the Canadian
memorial Chiropractic College and of Los Angeles College of
Chiropractic, in his book *The Neurodynamics of the Vertebral
Subluxation*, first published in 1963, brought together the
thoughts and experimental work of anatomists, physiologists,
neurologists, medical practitioners and chiropractors in an
attempt at explaining the nature and the effects of the lesion
known to chiropractors as a subluxation. Professor C. H. Suh,

a specialist in Biomechanics at the University of Colorado, has used computer-aided X-ray analysis and three-dimensional computer graphics, to study the biomechanical effects of chiropractic adjustments. This work started in the 1960's and is still continuing.

## Motion Palpation

One of the greatest contributions to chiropractic came from Henri Gillet, a recently retired chiropractor from Brussels, Belgium, and his colleague M. Liekens. Gillet's book *Belgian Chiropractic Reasearch Notes* may not be considered research in the sense in which most people think of it. The son of a chiropractor, he could not stand the empirical use of adjustment simply because it worked. He studied exactly what a subluxation was, and came to the conclusion that it was a disorder of movement. He has spent the last forty or more years observing first the normal movements between vertebrae, then the abnormal, and their effects and correction. He put common sense into chiropractic. What is more, he used no instrumentation. He simply used his hands, not only to treat, but also with his eyes as the instruments of his research.

## Undergraduate Research

In the third and fourth years of their study course, the students at the Anglo-European College of Chiropractic in Bournemouth work on a thesis which is presented as part of their final examination. Students review the literature on some aspect of chiropractic and undertake an experimental research project. Thus the fundamental importance of research is brought home to the chiropractic students, not only to make them evaluate critically what they study, but in the hope that they may contribute, through further research in the future, to the body of knowledge. Chiropractors of the future will by this means be enabled to produce scientific evidence for their assertions and no longer be regarded as an 'unscientific cult'. Other colleges are following the example of the AECC.

## Clinical Trials

One form of research which seems an obvious necessity is a controlled trial, comparing chiropractic with other methods of treatment, particularly in back pain, for which at least 50 per cent of patients consult a chiropractor. Various trials have been carried out but none has been really satisfactory for a number of reasons. First, we should compare chiropractic treatment with no treatment. It is, after all, often said that patients get better in spite of treatment. Secondly, in order to select the patients for the trial, there needs to be an agreed diagnosis. Chiropractors often make a spinal analysis without giving the patient's condition a label which is an accepted medical diagnosis. The diagnosis of low back pain is in any case notoriously vague. Thirdly, the observers who examine the patients before and after treatment should not know which patients have been assigned to be treated with chiropractic and which to non-treatment. Neither must the patients be told whether they are receiving chiropractic adjustments or no treatment. This is the essence of a double blind trial. It is amazing how difficult it is to perform a manipulation which, whilst fooling the patient into thinking he has been treated, is not likely to produce any alteration in the patient's physical condition. Trials designed to compare chiropractic with medical, physiotherapy and other treatments are even more difficult to devise. Dummy pills are easy to produce, but dummy chiropractic or dummy physiotherapy is not.

## British Chiropractic Association Trials

A. C. Breen collected information from forty-nine chiropractors between October 1973 and 1974 in a retrospective trial designed to identify the patient population, the complaints presented to chiropractors, and the type and duration of treatment. Just over 50 per cent of patients had low back pain, of which 96 per cent improved. The average number of treatment sessions to optimum benefit was seven, but just under 20 per cent of patients needed between eleven and forty attendances. It showed that one should not despair if little improvement had occurred after seven or more adjustments, because improvement was still possible. There was an almost equal ratio of male to female patients. They tended to be middle class and between 35 and 65 years old.

At present under way is a controlled trial of chiropractic and hospital outpatient treatment in association with the Medical Research Council. The trial entered the planning stage in 1982. A feasibility study funded by the Medical Research Council's Epidemiology and Medical Care Unit at Northwick Park, Harrow, England, has been completed and the results were published in the *Journal of Epidemiology and Community Health* in March 1986. They showed that such a trial was possible. Ten centres have been nominated to take part in the main trial. Each consists of a chiropractic practice and a hospital outpatient department. Patients will be allocated randomly to either and they will be assessed through questionnaires. The trial will, it is hoped, give some indication as to how effective chiropractic is in terms of disability and pain when compared with 'orthodox' hospital outpatient procedures.

There is no doubt that much research needs to be done. One of the main problems is finance. Chiropractic colleges have tended to be independently financed, as is the case with the AECC. Money for research is hard to come by. Recognition of the chiropractic course as a degree course may lead to attachment of chiropractic colleges to universities, thus opening them up to receiving government money. If the chiropractors themselves no longer have to support their own colleges financially, more money may become available to support much-needed research.

## The Test of Time

Aspirin and other drugs were swallowed by the ton long before proof of their mechanisms of action were available, because the clinical proof of relief of symptoms was thought to be sufficient. Electric convulsive therapy (ECT) is used on patients with chronic depression because it works, even though the mechanism of action is poorly understood. We should of course keep trying to understand, to experiment, to prove the truth beyond doubt. But it is not necessary to prove beyond question and to understand every detail of how and why a treatment works before it can be used. If it is successful, we can be sure that we shall continue to learn and understand more and more with the passage of time. And this is happening with chiropractic.

Chiropractic has now ninety-one years of clinical results. Its success in treating neuromusculoskeletal conditions is indisputable, and for back pain its record is second to none. The principal objection raised against it is that it is based on a philosophy that a vertebral subluxation is the cause of all disease. That hypothesis can safely be discarded without destroying chiropractic.

Since the 1970's when the General Medical Council relaxed its objections to registered medical practitioners collaborating with other (non-medical) health care workers, co-operation between chiropractors and doctors has increased. A trial such as has been described above, effected with the help of the Medical Research Council, would not have been possible twenty years ago. Younger doctors in particular have adopted therapies which were not taught to them in medical school, finding in them something which was lacking in the orthodox approach. Hypnotherapy, accupuncture and homoeopathy as well as spinal manipulative therapy of one form or another have been adopted by many general practitioners.

The increasing popularity of so-called alternative therapies with doctors has only reflected a growing awareness amongst the general public that orthodox medicine is not the only avenue to be explored in the search for health. Prince Charles, in his inaugural address as President of the British Medical Association in 1982, reflected this point of view by suggesting that there was a need for doctors to be open-minded in assessing therapies outside their field of competence and to be more willing to examine alternatives.

It is in this climate of open-mindedness that chiropractic has received more publicity through the media. Articles on chiropractic have appeared in recent years in many newspapers and magazines, there have been programmes about it on radio and on television, and chiropractors have been mentioned in chat shows, plays and even in strip cartoons. Furthermore, the medical press has also featured articles on chiropractic. In short, chiropractic is fast becoming an accepted method of treatment, especially for back pain.

Back pain has of course become a universal problem. In our sedentary, overweight society, which otherwise enjoys good health, back pain has acquired greater prominence. According to Philip Wood of the Arthritis and Rheumatism Council Epidemiology Research Unit, of Manchester University, over a million people in Great Britain consult their GP with back pain in any one year. Of those suffering disability from back pain, one in five is disabled severely enough to be unable to work. Two out of five have to change their job, and the remaining two are limited in the kind or amount of work they can do.

Few people can be unaware of what back pain feels like. A rapidly effective and inexpensive way of overcoming back pain is sought at some time by nearly every one of us. Chiropractic provides an answer.

## Chapter 4

# Benefits

**Vertebragenous Diseases**

The term vertebragenous is used to denote diseases arising from the vertebral column. Some use the word vertebrogenic but since this word gives the impression that the disease gives rise to the vertebrae and not the other way around (cf glucogenic, osteogenic) it is best avoided. A large section of such diseases is the low back pain group, the lumbago-sciaticas. Most of these are due to injury to the intervertebral disc caused either by a particular trauma or by a succession of minor traumata of which the patient may be unaware. They are associated with mechanical dysfunction in the spine, particularly with fixation of intervertebral joints. There are of course other causes of back pain, some of these are serious, such as secondary cancer, a bone cancer called myeloma and tuberculosis of bone, which must be excluded but which are relatively rare. Similar problems occur in the neck, producing neck pain, and pain referred to the shoulder and arm (cervico-brachialgia). In many cases there may be prolapse of the disc nucleus in the low back or excrescences from the disc together with osteophytes in the neck causing nerve root symptoms. Restoration of normal movement to the vertebral column will often relieve the nerve root pressure. If not, by taking abnormal strain off the disc it will allow regression of the swollen or displaced disc tissue. Even osteophytes, those little spurs of bone associated with degenerative disc disease, have been known to shrink once normal mechanical function has been restored. So we include the prolapsed lumbar discs, cervical disc lesions and cervical spondylosis as treatable by chiropractic. Similarly, chest pains not due to heart disease, lung disease or oesophagitis (inflammation of the oesophagus or gullet) or shingles, often come from disturbed spinal mechanics in the thoracic (dorsal) spine. Again, headaches are frequently 'mechanical'. Even true migraines often have as at least part of their cause cervical intervertebral joint dysfunction. Dizziness, vertigo and loss of balance are very often due to abnormalities of mobility in the cervical spine. If it is remembered that all the spinal nerves supply spinal joints, and that irritation of these nerves at the level of the joints can cause referred pain in whatever part of the body is supplied by the same nerve, it is obvious that spinal joint pain can be felt anywhere in the body. Conversely, among the differential diagnoses of a pain anywhere in the body, must be vertebragenous pain. In many cases it is the commonest cause of such pain, but is often the last one to be thought of.

The above diseases are described in the *Report of the Commission of Inquiry on Chiropractic in New Zealand*, 1979, as type M diseases. It lists a series of 'organic' diseases which chiropractors have claimed to help as type 0. They range from allergy to warts and the idea that some of them can be helped by manipulating the spine seems far-fetched. One must realize, however, that if chiropractic treatment is given to a patient with asthma, it may help the mobility of the patient's chest. Patients with Parkinson's disease may benefit from relieving intervertebral joint dysfunction, which is associated with the loss of co-ordination and may be making things worse. Similarly, no chiropractor ever cured multiple sclerosis, but chiropractic may be part of the treatment and help to relieve pain due to muscle spasms and pain which is not directly due to the disease. Even patients with cancers may benefit from spinal manipulative therapy, not to cure the cancer, but to cure other symptoms which may be associated or co-incidental. One of the 'ailments' listed as treated by chiropractic in the New Zealand Report is pregnancy. Clearly, pregnancy is not an ailment, but symptoms occurring in pregnancy, such as back pain due to change in posture, hormonal changes in the ligaments, and disc lesions, are amenable to chiropractic treatment. I would certainly not dispute the fact that improvements in the functioning of internal organs happened once spinal mobility is restored. I myself believe that functional problems such as 'spastic colon' in which the large bowel seems to tighten up and can be felt like a cord in the abdomen, is helped by chiropractic. Irritation of nerve endings in the intervertebral joints, as well as irritation of the spinal nerves themselves may well have secondary effects on the autonomic nerves controlling the muscular wall of the bowel. If we accept that psychogenic factors may affect such function, then why not mechanical factors sending noxious impulses into the central nervous system?

There are two reasons why the early chiropractors may have thought they had hit on a treatment for the cause of all disease. The first is that common things are commonest, and there are no diseases more common than those associated with intervertebral joint dysfunction. So, just as a broad spectrum antibiotic is more likely to cure an unknown infection than one which only attacks one type of bacterium, so a treatment which helps many diseases is more likely to help a disease of uncertain origin than a treatment which only helps a rare condition. The second reason is that diagnosis was less accurate at the turn of the century than it is in the latter half of the twentieth century. Just think what modern medical technology has done to make diagnosis more scientific and more accurate. Vertebragenous symptoms are great mimics. Thus a pain in the centre of the chest on exertion may be angina pectoris, but it may be referred from the spine. Similarly, pain in the upper abdomen may be due to an ulcer, but ulcer pain has to be differentiated from pain from the lower thoracic spine. A patient with such a condition may receive treatment for the wrong problem, then go to a chiropractor and be treated correctly. No wonder the early chiropractors could cure patients with all sorts of medical diagnoses. Many were obviously misdiagnoses. It is important to realize that if a patient has a chest pain and appropriate tests are carried out to exclude angina, it is not sufficient to tell the patient that he has not got angina. If his chest pain is of any severity he wants to get rid of it. The correct diagnosis should be made and the correct treatment instituted. The correct treatment for vertebragenous pain in most cases is vertebral adjustment.

## Rheumatism

As already discussed, chiropractic is very much concerned with painful conditions. Many of these painful conditions become more frequent in middle age, when there is some degenerative change in the joints of the body and in the discs. This group of diseases is often referred to as rheumatism. Many chiropractic patients wear copper bracelets which are said to prevent 'rheumatism'. The word should be avoided. To the doctor, it usually means rheumatic fever (acute rheumatism) or rheumatoid arthritis (chronic rheumatism). To a layman, it may be reassuring: 'It's only rheumatism', or it may conjure up thoughts of incurable pain.

Fibrositis is a term frequently used for tender areas in muscles associated with nodules and trigger spots. It is really a referred tenderness, the cause being found in the spine. Thus tender nodules in the trapezius muscles are associated with dysfunction in the joints of the neck, and tenderness in the upper part of the buttock with lumbar spinal lesions. Once the spinal mechanics are corrected, the muscle tenderness disappears. There is no doubt, however, that relief can also be obtained by pressure on the tender spots. Fibrositis, then, is another condition amenable to chiropractic, but is again a vague term which does not denote a definite pathology, and can therefore mean different things to different people.

## Postural Abnormalities

Abnormal spinal curvatures such as lumbar lordosis (sway back), thoracic kyphosis (round shoulders) and scoliosis (sideways curvature, sometimes with a rib hump or hunchback) can be helped by chiropractic. The gradual bending forward of the head with prominence of the lower neck and upper thoracic vertebrae (the dowager's hump) is another example of postural deformity. Once they have been present for a long time, such conditions may not be correctable, or may be only partially so. The most effective way of preventing deterioration and reducing to some extent the deformities is by restoring normal mobility to the joints. Once an abnormal curve begins to form, the stresses on the spinal joints cause fixations — that is, loss of mobility between adjacent vertebrae — to occur, increasing the deformity. Regeneration of discs, though it occurs to some extent, is a very slow process indeed as cartilage has no blood supply. Once a disc has thinned or become wedge-shaped, it can be helped to regain its shape by re-introducing movement into the joints which have become fixed. Restoration of mobility helps to stimulate regeneration, but the improvement is likely not to be complete.

## Prevention

From what has been said about incomplete recovery from degenerative conditions, it can be seen that prevention is important. Here, chiropractic has a place. By restoring normal mobility to joints and correcting the posture and mechanical function of the spine as a whole, abnormal stresses leading to degeneration are prevented. Degenerative change occurs in cartilage either because of excessive stress (for instance, shearing forces causing tearing and fissures in intervertebral discs), or because of absence of movement leading to atrophy (wasting due to lack of nourishment) as cartilage, having no blood supply, depends on movement for exchange of fluids and nutrients to take place.

Because degenerative changes happen over a prolonged period, and the changes showing on X-ray films appear slowly, it is difficult to demonstrate the preventative effect of chiropractic on these conditions. Regeneration occurs even more slowly, so improvement sufficient to be visible on X-ray films is not often seen. Improvement in the posture and well-being of the patient are frequently noticeable, however, and the arresting of a progressive degenerative process is often observed. In common with many chiropractors, I have no doubt that chiropractic care of the spine prevents and even reverses degenerative change in intervertebral joints including the discs.

## Accessory Treatments

There is no reason why chiropractic treatment should be an alternative to other therapies. Physiotherapists use ultrasonics, interferential therapy, massage, heat and ice. These can usually be combined with spinal manipulative therapy and indeed are used by some chiropractors themselves.

Similarly, when prolapsed lumbar discs fail to respond to chiropractic, there may be a large disc bulge. Nerve root inflammation and swelling can often be reduced by an epidural injection of local anaesthetic. A very large disc protrusion interfering with a nerve root can be an indication for disc surgery. There is no reason why chiropractic treatment may not be used to resolve residual symptoms after either of these procedures. If the disc protrusion is still present for instance, in a case requiring epidural injection the chiropractor will of course need to be careful not to use a manipulation which may put pressure on the disc and increase the protrusion. These treatments are not mutually exclusive, however. Even traction can be used at the same time as manipulation. I consider traction to be a very non-specific form of manipulation, however. If chiropractic adjustments alone are not helping, I should not expect traction to have much effect.

Chiropractic is traditionally a drugless therapy. There is, however, no reason why drugs may not be used in conjunction with chiropractic. In the painful stage of any condition, painkillers, such as Paracetamol/Codeine preparations can be of great benefit in making the patient more comfortable while healing is taking place. Similarly, muscle relaxants, although on the whole not very effective, have their place, as do hypnotics to help the patient get some sleep, and even occasionally corticosteroid injections, although these should be used with caution as they interfere with the body's healing processes, which the chiropractor is usually trying to stimulate. In the acute stage of a prolapsed disc, an injection of a powerful painkiller such as pethidine may be essential before any other treatment, even moving the patient to bed, can be undertaken.

While on the subject of drugs, it should be mentioned that the chiropractor ought to be aware of what medicines the patient is taking. Not only may some symptoms be caused by drugs, but certain drugs — for instance, anticoagulants — are indications for caution with manipulation, which could cause bruising or even haemorrhage into joints. Other treatments, whether for the condition for which the chiropractor was consulted or for another condition, may require modification in the treatment programme. As in all fields of medicine, co-operation and communication between all the practitioners treating a patient is essential.

## Individual Variations

Every treatment suits some patients better than others, and chiropractic is no exception. Just as some patients are unusually afraid of injections, some may have an inordinate fear of being manipulated. A chiropratic adjustment at its best is gentle, quick and painless. Nervous tension on the part of the patient can make it difficult, even with a rapid adjustment, since muscular relaxation is essential. A skilled chiropractor can overcome this problem. Knowing how to make the patient relax is part of his art. Furthermore he can feel when the patient is 'off-guard' and make use of the moment. Similarly, to relax is the best way to allow a manipulation to have its effect. If the patient holds himself tense, the restoration of normal muscle tone may be prevented.

All treatment is influenced by the state of mind of the patient, and improvement is less likely to occur if the patient does not believe he will improve, or even worse if he does not want to. A confident relaxed attitude on the part of the chiropractor is important. Painful manipulations are on the whole useless, and frighten the patient. Fear on the part of the patient is the greatest impediment to effective treatment. So a trusting patient, and a confident skilful chiropractor who can administer a rapid painless adjustment in a relaxed manner, is an ideal recipe for success.

*Chapter 5*

# How Do I Find a Chiropractor?

**Referral**

Increasing numbers of general practitioners are referring patients to chiropractors practising in their area. This is the ideal way. In Britain we are lucky to have a primary health care system in which the general practitioner is the key figure. When a person is in need of any kind of medical care, he first approaches his GP. Many matters are dealt with by the GP himself, but should he feel a specialist's opinion or a particular type of therapist is indicated, he will refer the patient to him. His choice of therapist or consultant is made not only through his knowledge of medical science and of the facilities available, but also from his personal knowledge of the individuals involved, both doctors or therapists and patient. He is thus able to choose the right man or woman to whom to refer a particular patient for a particular problem. It also means that the consultant or therapist will communicate his findings and/or treatment to the GP, so that a comprehensive medical record is kept by the GP.

Chiropractors, unless they are also medically qualified, do not necessarily insist on a referral from the patient's general practitioner. It is, as we have seen only in recent years that doctors have been permitted by the General Medical Council in this country to refer patients to chiropractors at all. There are a few chiropractors who are also medically qualified. They are rare, however, because unlike the osteopathic profession, which has the London College of Osteopathic Medicine to train medical doctors in osteopathy, there are at present in this country no facilities for training doctors in chiropractic except through the standard four-year course at the Anglo-European College of Chiropractic in Bournemouth. Many patients therefore approach a chiropractor through the recommendation of friends or members of their family who have themselves received chiropractic treatment. Patients are keen to pass on to others the name of someone who has helped them. How else can anybody decide who is good at his job except through recommendation? Several recommendations will often convince a patient that a particular chiropractor is worth consulting.

There are of course indications, such as the qualifications of the practitioner, that he has attended a recognized course of training, and that he is accepted within the profession. It is important to check the standing of the chiropractor, because in Britain at present, unlike the USA, Canada, Australia, New Zealand and Switzerland, there is no official registration by the State. This means that anyone, with or without proper training, can call themselves a chiropractor. The best way to be sure of his credentials is to consult a member of the British Chiropractic Association. It is true that some chiropractors who may be eligible to join the association choose not to do so, but most do, and membership acts as a guarantee that they have the recognition of the profession.

## The British Chiropractic Association
This association accepts as members graduates of the Anglo-European College of Chiropractic and of colleges accredited by the Council on Chiropractic Education of the United States. Members agree to abide by its rules and byelaws and to its code of ethics which regulates the relationships between chiropractors, between chiropractors and other professions and between the chiropractor and his patients. Complaints against individual chiropractors are investigated by a disciplinary committee who may reprimand, impose fines or remove the member's name from the register. It publishes a register of names, addresses and telephone numbers of members which is revised annually.

As well as regulating the profession and uniting it, the British Chiropractic Association provides spokesmen to represent the profession for the media and for discussions with other health professionals, and works for improvement in public relations for chiropractic. It runs postgraduate courses and bi-annual conferences to keep members in touch with developments in both chiropractic and medical subjects. It promotes research into chiropractic, and it supports the Anglo-European College of Chiropractic in every possible way, including giving financial assistance. It is affiliated to the European Chiropractors' Union, which brings together ten national associations and publishes a quarterly journal.

## Fees

Chiropractic is unfortunately not available under the National Health Service. Members charge fees for services which vary in different parts of the country, but tend to be lower than the fees for private medical consultations. There may be additional charges for the initial examination and for X-rays. Unless the chiropractor is medically qualified he is not exempt from value added tax, so part of his charges are to cover this. Many of the provident associations and private medical insurances are still refusing to reimburse chiropractors' fees unless the patient is referred to him by a hospital consultant.

Obtaining the services of a chiropractor may still require some effort, and perhaps the willingness to travel some distance, as not all of Britain is adequately provided for. Chiropractors become thinner on the ground as you travel north. It is expensive, in that the total cost must be borne by the patient, and even private medical insurance may fail to cover it. People are realizing more and more, however, the importance of looking after their bodies, and the need to put money into keeping fit. Those who do so usually find that health is a very good investment.

## Chapter 6

# What Can I Expect When I go For Treatment?

Just as counselling is about listening, so chiropractic is about touching and feeling (palpation). Like any doctor, the chiropractor starts by conducting an interview with the patient (history taking), in which he will learn the patient's symptoms and their severity and duration and pattern of occurrence. He will also ask about his past illnesses and previous treatment, occupation and any other relevant details.

He conducts a general examination for which a male patient is stripped to his underpants and a female patient is provided with a gown which is open at the back. He pays particular reference to the nervous system and goes through the standard orthopaedic tests, such as the straight leg-raising test with the patient lying on his back, in low back complaints. With the patient erect, he makes an assessment of the patient's posture, including the arches of the feet, leg length, pelvic tilt, abnormal curvatures of the spine and any kinks or distortions. The sense which is most important to the chiropractor is that of touch. From the first day at chiropractic college he learns to feel the backs and necks of his fellow students, to feel what is normal, to touch, to palpate. The art of palpation, examination by touch, is the art of chiropractic. Static palpation is best carried out with the patient face-down, and most chiropractic couches are designed with a split headpiece so that patients can lie prone with their cheeks against cushions and their nose and mouth free. From static palpation the chiropractor assesses position, size, shape, resistance, tone, temperature and texture of the structures beneath his fingers, which include skin, fat, connective tissue, muscles, bones and joints. Tenderness is also observed from the reaction of the patient to gentle pressure.

Motion palpation (the assessment of mobility at intervertebral motor units, with the moving done by the examiner) is best carried out with the patient sitting. This may be done by feeling with the back of the right hand all the way up the patient's back with a series of gentle prods, while holding the patient's chin with the left hand. By this means the 'give' in the intervertebral joints is felt. When he arrives at the atlas — the upper vertebra of the spine, just below the base of the skull he takes it in a thumb and forefinger grasp, and presses it forwards, so that the play between the atlas and the occiput (base of the skull) can be assessed. The posterior joints of the neck vertebrae form a pillar on each side of the midline. These articular pillars, as they are called, are felt by the fingers of one hand, as the neck is moved in each direction in turn — that is, in flexion and extension, in sideways flexion and in rotation, by the other hand on the patient's head. The spinous processes of the vertebrae are palpable as the knobs down the centre of the back. By placing a finger alongside adjacent spinous processes and moving the thoracic and lumbar spines into flexion and extension, lateral flexion in either direction and rotation, through an arm placed across the front or the back of the patient's shoulders, abnormalities of movement can be felt in the intervertebral joints of these areas. Again, more accurate observation of lumbar joints and the sacro-iliac joints at the posterior aspect of the pelvis can be obtained by grasping the ilium (hip bone) with one hand with the thumb at the back and placing the thumb of the other hand on the lumbar spinous processes and on the sacrum in turn, meanwhile asking the patient to raise his knees up to his chest. Movement, normal or impaired, between the thumbs reflects the lumbar intervertebral and sacro-iliac movement. It can be appreciated both by feel and by vision.

As well as making a diagnosis and deciding whether the patient's complaint is due to mechanical abnormalities in the spine or to an organic disease, the important thing which has been learned in the examination of the patient by the chiropractor is which particular joints have impaired mobility. It is these which are susceptible to manipulative correction.

The chiropractor may require to take X-rays of the patient's spine. It may be, therefore, that he will postpone treatment until the second visit. Before commencing treatment, he must decide that chiropractic is appropriate. Otherwise he will usually refer the patient back to his own doctor.

## Manipulative Therapy

Once the joint fixations have beeen discovered by palpation, treatment is also manual. The basic chiropractic manipulation, usually referred to as an adjustment, is a sharp thrust applied across a joint in such a way as to separate the joint surfaces to snap the joint open. It is akin to cracking the knuckles, and the joint crack which is usually both heard and felt is the same. It is caused by the sudden separation of surfaces lined by flexible material (cartilage) and having a thin film of (synovial) fluid between them. A similar sound is produced by pulling a moist rubber sucker off a glass surface.

Methods of adjustment are many and varied. They are all methods of abruptly separating joint surfaces. The feature which characterizes chiropractic adjustment is the rapid thrust. One of the traditional methods of adjustment is called the toggle recoil adjustment. Contact is made against the bone to be moved with the pisiform region of the adjusting hand. The pisiform is the small bone protruding at the front of the wrist where it joins the palm above the little finger. The wrist of the adjusting hand is gripped by the other hand. The shoulders are positioned directly above the bone to be adjusted, and the arrangement of the shoulders elbows and wrists is such that the elbows act as toggles, the sudden straightening of which produces a rapid thrust at the point of contact and immediate recoil. This adjustment can be used almost anywhere in the spine and has been traditionally a popular method of adjusting the upper cervical vertebrae.

Most of the thoracic joints can be adjusted by using a contact

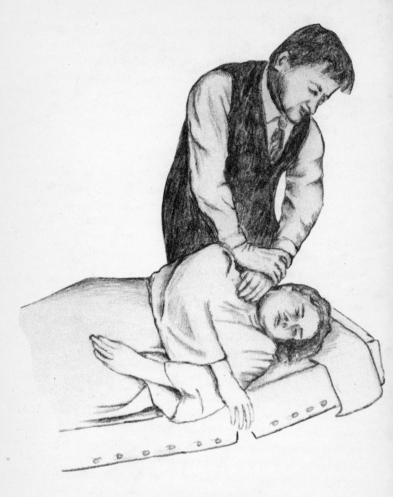

Figure 8    Toggle Recoil Adjustment

on either side of the column of spinous processes at the back of the chest with either the ulnar (little finger) border of the hand or the thenar eminences (at the base of the thumbs). A little headward pressure is used to 'take up the slack' in the soft

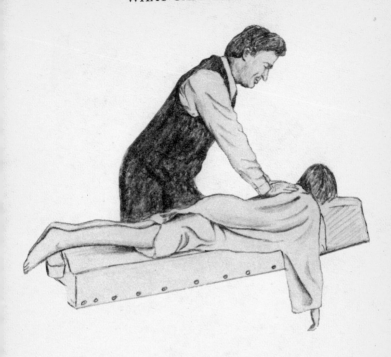

Figure 9   Adjusting the Thoracic Spine

tissues and in the joints and then a sudden downward thrust is applied. Cracks are usually heard as the joints beneath the contacts are forced open.

In the lumbar region, the roll position can be used. The patient is placed on his side with his upper knee bent and his foot hooked behind the lower knee. His shoulders are rotated so that he is almost lying on his back with the upper half of his body. The upper shoulder is stabilized with one hand, whilst the adjusting hand contacts just to the upper side of the spinous process of the lumbar vertebra to be moved. Thus contact on L5 (the fifth lumbar vertebra) will move the L4-5 joint. A sudden thrust towards the patient's abdomen causes the posterior joint on that side to snap open. A similar position may

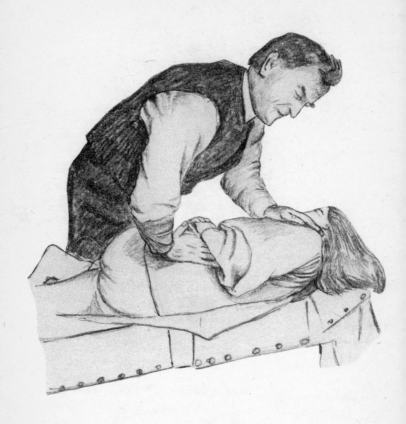

Figure 10    A Lumbar Adjustment

be used to adjust the sacro-iliac joints by contacting the sacrum
to move it on the lower ilium (the hip bone), or contacting the
upper ilium to move it on the sacrum.

We will see later that there are different schools, systems and
variations of chiropractic technique. Its distinctive features are
nevertheless assessment of abnormalities of vertebral mechanics
by palpation, and manual correction using rapid thrust
adjustment.

## Length of Treatment

The initial examination may take 20-45 minutes, or more if X-ray films are taken. Follow-up visits do not normally take more than 10-20 minutes but obviously the amount of time necessary varies according to the needs of the patient and his problem. Again, the interval between treatments is a matter for deciding in each particular case. The interval can be anything from one day upwards. Probably weekly sessions are suitable in the average case. A little time is necessary for each adjustment to be fully effective. Follow-up sessions may be necessary, especially in longstanding or habitual problems at anything from a few weeks to a year. After a course of treatment, any recurrence of symptoms should be dealt with immediately as it can often be corrected in a much shorter time.

The number of treatment sessions necessary varies greatly. An average patient may require between six and ten visits. Longstanding problems and patients with marked degenerative disease are likely to take longer than problems of recent onset where the spine is in good condition.

After an adjustment, the patient is usually aware that something has happened. Sometimes improvement is immediate. Sometimes half a dozen sessions are necessary before improvement is noticed. Chiropractic treatment is not normally painful, unless the patient is in pain at the time, so that touching causes pain. Patients are often surprised to find it is painless. However, painful reactions do occur, especially after the first treatment. This may consist of soreness or stiffness or occasionally more severe pain. It usually means that the treatment is taking effect. Joints that were not moving are now moving and initially are causing symptoms. Such reactions can be dealt with by simple explanation, rest, and/or mild or rarely strong painkillers. They subside within 24-48 hours and should not be a cause for alarm.

## Auxiliary Diagnostic Methods

As well as palpation, various pieces of apparatus can be used to assist chiropractic analysis and diagnosis, and all kinds of investigations may be performed. They are used more or less often by different chiropractors. Some are specific to chiropractic. Others are commonly used in medical practice.

## Posturometry

Since posture and body mechanics are closely associated, chiropractors have always been concerned with variations from the ideal posture, and the stresses on the spine caused thereby. A simple traditional method of analyzing posture is the plumb line. From the back, an imaginery line dropped vertically from the prominence at the base of the skull, known as the external occipital protuberance, should pass through the gluteal cleft between the buttocks, and hit the floor between the feet. From the side, a line dropped vertically from the external auditory meatus (the ear hole) should pass through the hip, behind the kneecap, and hit the floor in front of the ankle. More complicated versions of grids and posturometers are sometimes used to measure skeletal distortions, pelvic tilt and scoliosis (spinal curvature).

Correctness of posture may also be assessed from the distribution of weight on the feet. The patient may be made to stand on a pair of scales to measure the evenness of the weight distribution on each foot. Split scales can even measure the distribution of weight between the forefoot and the heels on each side. Motorized treadmills are sometimes used to assess normality of the gait, and pelvic movements.

## Radiography

The majority of chiropractors either have their own radiographic apparatus, or have access to diagnostic radiology facilities. X-ray films taken with the patient standing are useful in assessing posture and abnormality of the spinal curves. The antero-posterior curves show on the lateral view. A sideways curvature or twist of the spine, known as scoliosis, shows in the antero-posterior view, and the amount of sideways bending or the radius of the curve can be measured. If the radiograph is taken with the X-ray beam centred at the level of the hip joints, and the patient is standing with his legs straight and his feet slightly apart, then any difference in leg length can be measured.

Minute measurements of vertebral misalignments are sometimes made by drawing lines on X-ray films, and measuring distances between bony points on either side of the spine. X-ray measurements can be very useful diagnostically, but asymmetries in the human body abound, and that fact, combined with the distortion inherent in the technique of projecting an X-ray beam on to a film with the object at a distance from it, make exaggerated use of such measurements unrewarding.

One way in which subluxations and intervertebral fixations can be seen radiologically, is by taking views in different positions — for instance, lateral views of the neck with patient's chin on his chest, and then with his head bent backwards (flexion and extension views). These show whether normal movement has taken place at each intervertebral segment. Similarly, antero-posterior views can be taken in sidebending. Cineradiography, the taking of moving radiographs which can be preserved on film or videotape, can be quite enlightening in showing impaired or excessive movement at different levels of the spine, but is expensive and can require high levels of exposure to X-radiation. It is beyond the reach of the average chiropractor.

The disadvantage of depending too much on X-ray films to diagnose subluxations is the changing pattern of fixations which occurs from one visit to the next, particularly when the patient is adjusted. It would in theory require a repeat X-ray at each visit to the chiropractor to assess the current position.

X-rays are of great importance in screening for pathology. Spinal tumours such as multiple myeloma, secondary cancer deposits and Hogkin's disease can be detected. Bony infections (osteomyelitis) and infective arthritis are recognizable from their X-ray appearances. Fractures, dislocations, generalized thinning of bone in osteoporosis or osteomalacea, all these are important to anyone who is intending to apply sudden force to the spine. X-rays also show up congenital fusions (in which joints are absent from birth) and asymmetries as well as surgical fusions. Degenerative disease of discs and spinal joints shows as narrowing of disc and joint spaces and formation of bony outgrowths known as osteophytes.

Some conditions seen on X-ray will be contra-indications for manipulation, or may be indications for care or avoidance of particular techniques. Others will suggest a completely different form of therapy or referral to the appropriate specialist. All in all, radiography is an exceedingly useful tool for the chiropractor, but should be used selectively as excessive amounts of radiation are known to be harmful. X-rays should be avoided altogether in some circumstances such as early pregnancy.

Diagnostic radiology has expanded considerably in recent years. Techniques such as tomography, computerized tomography, ultrasonic scanning, radioisotope scanning and nuclear magnetic resonance can all be useful in evaluating spinal pathology and congenital or acquired abnormalities. Such techniques, however, require referral to specialized units.

## Blood and Urine Tests

Laboratory tests also play their part in diagnosis of bone disease, infections and rheumatic diseases. Chiropractors usually have access to pathological laboratories either directly or indirectly by referral through the patient's general practitioner. Only simple tests can be performed in a small clinic, but the ESR or erythrocyte sedimentation rate, which is done on a sample of blood removed by syringe from a vein, and urine tests for blood, protein and sugar are carried out in many chiropractic clinics. The ESR is useful in screening for a variety of inflammatory diseases, and particularly rheumatoid arthritis, ankylosing spondylitis and polymyalgia rheumatica, which are commonly seen in chiropractic practice. It can warn the chiropractor that the problem is not a simple mechanical one.

## The Neurocalometer

In the early days of chiropractic, it was thought that when a bone impinged on a nerve, it produced a state of excitability, and therefore heat. Indeed, a characteristic of disease was said to be inflammation, and the heat produced was supposedly produced by excessive nerve force due to irritation of the nerve supplying the organ. One way of looking for a state of excitability in the spinal nerves was to look for increased heat production. The Palmer School of Chiropractic produced an instrument which measured small variations in temperature on either side of the spinal column. It consisted of a pair of thermocouples, like two prongs, attached to a meter with a needle which swung to the right or left according to which side of the spine the temperature was highest. A more sophisticated piece of equipment was known as the neurocalograph. This recorded the differential temperatures on opposite sides of the spine on a roll of graph paper. After allowing a few seconds for the meter to stabilize, with the probes of the instrument in position at the base of the skull, the instument was moved at a regular pace down the spine to the coccyx of the seated patient. Some instruments were motorized to assist this steady motion down the patient's back. A tracing was produced showing deviations on either side of the vertical, indicating discrepancies in the temperature on either side of the spine, which were said to be due to subluxations. The nearer the tracing was to a straight line, the healthier the patient. Correct adjustments of vertebrae were expected to iron out the deviations on the neurocalograph tracing.

Such instruments still exist and are used, although not extensively. Some have only one probe to measure hot spots and cold spots. Prolapsed discs often produce areas of vasodilatation or increased skin blood flow, and therefore heat, while tender areas in muscles are frequently found to have reduced temperature due to constriction of the small blood vessels.

Those who used neurocalometers were often of the HIO (Hole-in-one) school, who adjusted the atlas (the uppermost

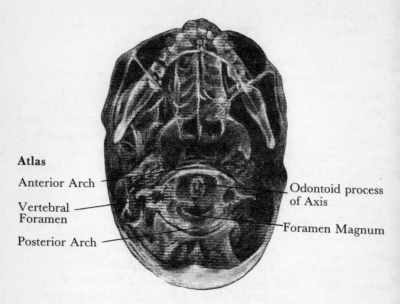

Atlas

Anterior Arch

Vertebral
Foramen

Posterior Arch

Odontoid process
of Axis

Foramen Magnum

Figure 11    The Vertex View

vertebra of the neck) almost invariably, whatever the condition being treated. A series of X-rays were taken which included the vertex view, in which the X-ray beam was projected through the skull from beneath the chin to the top of the head. This view allowed the vertebral foramen of the atlas, which encases the spinal cord, to be visualized superimposed on the foramen magnum, which surrounds the origin of the cord at the base of the brain. By careful analysis of the films, minor displacements of the atlas were diagnosed, and the 'line of drive' necessary to adjust the atlas correctly was worked out. If only one adjustment was to be made, how was the chiropractor to know if and when it was necessary to repeat it? To take a new X-ray each visit would be hazardous for the patient because of the radiation involved. Here is where neurocalograph tracing was useful. It could be repeated after adjustment to see if a change had been effected, and again each time the patient was seen, so that when the abnormal pattern re-appeared, the chiropractor could once more perform the adjustment.

## Other Diagnostic Methods

In modern medicine, technology has greatly expanded the range of diagnostic tests. There are many and varied laboratory procedures in the fields of haematology, serology and chemical pathology, which help in the diagnosis of bone, joint, muscular and nervous disease which may concern the chiropractor. These will not be elaborated upon as they require referral to the appropriate laboratory, and are not specifically chiropractic. The expansion of radiology has been discussed. Similarly, specialized techniques of thermography are available, mapping out the relatively hot and cold zones of the body. Electromyography and nerve conduction studies are used to detect defective neuromuscular function. The rapid development of medical technology has made it all the more important for the chiropractor not to isolate himself from the main stream of medicine, so that all the diagnostic methods of modern medicine are available to him.

*Chapter 7*

# Variations in Technique

Although there is great uniformity in the profession, there has grown up a diversity of techniques, both of analysis and of treatment. Many of these are known by the names of the teachers who advocate them. It is not possible to look at all of these, but we will look at some of the better-known systems to illustrate how variable can be the approach to the the patient, the diagnosis and the treatment, the object being always to restore the spine to normality in order to restore the patient's health.

**Sacro-occipital Technique**
SOT as it is often called, is linked to the name of Major Bertrand De Jarnette (born 1899) of Nebraska, who qualified in chiropractic at Nebraska College of Chiropractic in 1925. It is based on the fact that abnormal muscle tension around the pelvis affects the muscle tension in the top of the neck. When the sacrum moves in an abnormal direction, the atlas will move in an abnormal but opposite direction.

The patient is analysed according to his posture, apparent leg length (pelvic distortion causes one leg to appear longer than the other), and various tests known as the dollar sign, the crest sign, heel tension, the arm-fossa test and the SOT test. The tests used indicate excessive muscle tension and accompanying tenderness, muscle weakness, or distortions of the frame. The unusual feature of this technique, however, is the method of correction using blocks. The blocks are wedge-shaped, and measure 8 inches by 4 inches by 4 inches (20cm by 10cm by

10cm). They are padded, and placed under the upper or lower part of the pelvis with the patient lying on his back or front. Usually a block is placed under the upper part of the pelvis on one side and under the lower part on the other, thus producing a torsion with the patient's own body weight acting as the force of adjustment. It is a useful method of adjustment if the chiropractor does not wish to over-exert himself, or is not very strong.

## Gonstead

Clarence S. Gonstead (born 1898), a mechanical and automotive engineer, began his chiropractic career after recovery from acute rheumatoid arthritis. He graduated at Palmer College of Chiropractic in 1923, and at Minnesota Naturopathic College in 1943, and founded a large Health Care Centre at Mt Horeb, Wisconsin. His chiropractic methods are widely practised. An analysis of the patient is made with great emphasis on the X-ray film and lines drawn thereon to show distortions and misalignments. The pelvis, being the base on which the spine is built, is carefully analysed for tilts and rotations of the bones. Similarly, lines are drawn between corresponding points on either side of individual vertebrae and extended to show more clearly any disrelationship which exists between adjacent vertebrae. There can be anterior or posterior shift, rotation or wedging so that the gap between the vertebrae is wider on the right or on the left.

These abnormalities of position are said to be due to the disc. If the nucleus of the disc is displaced to the right, then the intervertebral space will be wider on the right than on the left, and so on. The object of adjustment is therefore to reposition the vertebra in such a way as to allow the nucleus of the disc to return to its normal position.

## Logan Basic Technique

Named after the late Hugh B. Logan, founder of Logan College of Chiropractic, Chesterfield, Missouri, in 1935, this technique relies on correcting the sacrum to affect the rest of the spine.

The *Textbook of Logan Basic Methods* states: 'The body of the lowest freely moveable vertebra always rotates towards the low side of the sacrum or the foundation upon which it rests, and rotates towards the high iliac crest when that crest is high as a result of sacral subluxation.' The most widely used technique of correcting the sacrum is known as the apex contact. The thumb is placed in the ischio-rectal fossa. This is the space between the rectum (the lower end of the bowel) and the ischium (that part of the pelvic bone on which one sits). Gentle pressure is made towards the head and upwards and sideways, and is held for about three minutes. The other hand meanwhile can make vibratory movements over the vertebrae or the muscles of the back. The contact is usually released suddenly.

The technique is said to cause relaxation, and is a useful preparatory treatment before other pelvic adjustments are made.

## Applied Kinesiology

George J. Goodheart (born 1918) of Detroit, Michigan, revived the use of reflexes described by an osteopath in the 1930's and known as Chapman's neurolymphatic reflexes. He also used neurovascular reflexes, previously described by another chiropractor, Terence Bennett. The former are points mainly adjacent to the spine and in the spaces between the ribs. They are stimulated by light rotary massage. The latter are mainly on the head and stimulated by very light touch. Goodheart found that these reflexes caused specific muscles, which were weak, to become stronger. Again, Goodheart associates specific muscle weaknesses with abnormal function of specific organs of the body. Other reflexes such as the meridians of acupuncture are also used.

An indicator muscle is used — for instance, the psoas, a large muscle which takes its origin in the abdomen from the lumbar vertebrae and is inserted into the femur (thigh bone) just below and internal to the hip joint. It can be tested by the patient's lifting the straight leg off the couch against resistance from the examiner. Applied kinesiologists state that it will become weak if the patient places his hands over a subluxated vertebra. Similarly, it will become weak if the patient places in his mouth a food to which he is 'allergic'. Removal of the cause or correction of the subluxation will restore the muscle to its full power. So will stimulation of the appropriate neurolymphatic or neurovascular reflex.

## Nimmo Technique

Raymond Nimmo was born in 1904 in Fort Worth, Texas, where he practised chiropractic from 1926 to 1956. He then moved to Granbury, Texas, and conducted seminars in his 'Receptor-Tonus' method all over the world during the 1970's. The Nimmo Technique, as it is called, is simpler still. It is common experience that if you have painful muscles, there are tender spots. These are areas of localized spasm in the muscles. Pressure on these trigger spots will produce muscular relaxation.

Patients with tender muscles often get great relief from the use of rotary massage on the 'nodules' in the muscles. According to Nimmo, it is unnecessary to use rotary massage. Simple pressure is even more effective.

## Lifts

Most chiropractors and indeed orthopaedic surgeons sometimes use heel lifts. If one leg is shorter than the other, then obviously the deformity can be corrected by increasing the heel of the shoe on the side of the short leg. If a fracture has caused the problem, then the shoe can be raised by the amount of shortening. When short legs have grown that way because of poliomyelitis in infancy or for no known reason, the body will have compensated, by permanent changes in the shape of bones, discs and joints, so that complete correction of the leg length would cause more trouble than it would solve. Only a fraction of the discrepancy is therefore added to the heel, half at the very most.

In many cases of scoliosis or sideways curvature of the spine, there is no actual leg length difference. Nevertheless, a heel lift may be used which will, by altering the tilt on the pelvis, tend to reduce the deformity. Of course, if much of a heel lift is used, one foot will tilt forwards more than the other, which can be uncomfortable. In this case, the sole and heel are raised.

Bilateral raised heels are sometimes used to increase the lordosis or hollow of the back. A heel raisé may also be used to take the strain off an injured Achilles tendon at the back of the ankle, or to alter the point of maximum pressure on the head of the femur in osteoarthritis of the hip. Raised soles, usually known as negative heels, are used to reduce the lumbar curve.

## Cranial Techniques

The bones of the skull are connected through joints called sutures. They are irregular very complicated saw-tooth arrangements and clearly permit very limited movement. The lower jaw or mandible articulates with the skull through a joint which is hinged and which glides forwards when the mouth is opened. Various movements are said to occur at the sutures of the skull. There is a fluctuation or wave-like motion, a respiratory motion, pulsation in time with that of the sinuses of the brain, and mandibular cranial motion (skull movement associated with jaw movements).

Of how much importance these skull movements are is difficult to say. Certainly, if there were no purpose in movement of these bones, there would be no joints. The function of the sutures and the anterior and posterior gaps in bones (fontanelles) in babies, is to allow compression and shaping of the skull during childbirth, so that the baby's head can pass through the birth canal. In the growing child, they permit growth and expansion of the brain. But in the fully grown man they fail to fuse, sometimes but by no means always doing so in old age. The norm throughout life is for some possibility of motion to remain in the skull sutures. The presumption is that there is movement between the bones that form the skull and that this movement has some purpose. Loss of mobility at these joints may therefore be expected to interfere with health in some way.

Cranial adjusting is not usually a rapid thrust procedure, but gentle pressure tending to correct immobility or malposition. Some of the cranial bones of the face are best mobilized with a finger in the mouth and some even use a finger in the nose.

## Motion Palpation

Henri Gillet, whose father Julius Gillet (died 1923) was the first chiropractor in Belgium, has already been mentioned in chapter 3. He must be given credit for the realization that the subluxation, the malposition which chiropractors had always sought to correct or adjust, was simply an abnormality of movement. Though distortions and misalignments could be seen on X-ray films, such films were static. The joints were not dislocated but within their normal range. The vertebrae were simply not moving in harmony with one another. He found that with careful examination of passive movement, that is, when the examiner forced movement into a particular joint, with the patient relaxed and allowing him to do so, some joints refused to move as they normally should. These places where he found joints immobile he termed 'fixations'.

Gillet divided such fixations into unifixes and bifixes, according to whether both paired posterior spinal joints were fixed, or just one of a pair, and into partial or complete fixations according to whether any movement at all was possible at those joints. He saw that the original cause of a fixation was spasm of the muscles moving the joint. Any joint injury is accompanied by splinting by the muscles which normally move the joint. Such splinting in the spinal joints is fixation. Splinting as a result of trauma or injury could be expected to be self-limiting. In fact, there is a tendency for spinal joints to remain fixed even after the initial cause has gone. Gillet explained this as due to intra-articular adhesion. In other words, the joint surfaces get 'stuck' together. It becomes evident when one adjusts such fixed joints that this happens, but the exact mechanism has not been fully demonstrated. Surgeons who have operated on 'frozen shoulders' have described the loss of mobility as being like the capsule of the joint adhering to the head of the humerus like a piece of Sellotape. Such adhesion is clearly different from the fibrous bands called adhesions in the abdomen after infections or surgery. It seems a stickiness of the synovia causes joint adhesion. The third more chronic or long-term type of fixation is restricted by shortened ligaments. Ligaments are passive and take the slack by shortening when there is no joint movement. When that has happened a joint may need adjusting a number of times to persuade it to move and cause the ligaments to regain normal length.

In motion palpation, the chiropractor not only feels the position of vertebrae relative to one another by feeling the parts of them which are accessible to his fingers, but he also forces movement into the joints he is palpating to assess the normality of passive movement. The passive movements felt can be either movements in the normal range of active motion or movement in a direction in which a person does not himself move the joint, the movement which is described as 'joint play'. The chiropractor can assess whether a joint is normal, fixed or excessively mobile.

An adjustment is a manipulation which removes or partially removes a fixation. It induces movement in the formerly fixed joint. It does not have to completely free the joint, as partial restoration of mobility will be completed by the forces of the body. Gillet also described 'fixation complexes' which were patterns of fixations tending to occur together. Restricted mobility in one part of the spine will have repercussions in other parts. So it is that one adjustment will often free a number of fixations. For this reason, and because other manipulations often caused irritation and worked in opposition to the first, he usually advocated performing only one adjustment at one session. A maxim which he adopted was 'find it, fix it, and leave it alone'. It is perhaps better stated 'find it, adjust it, and leave it alone'.

The idea of motion palpation as the basis of chiropractic has been spread in the USA by L. John Faye of The Motion Palpation Institute, in California.

## Listings

Static palpation of the spine and adjustments of misalignments involves describing the abnormal position of a vertebra. Thus the atlas is described on the basis of the position of the transverse processes which can be felt between the mastoid process and the angle of the jaw, just below the ear-lobe on either side. It is described as right posterior (RP) or left posterior (LP), right inferior (RI) or left inferior (LI), right lateral (RL), or left lateral (LL). Similarly, other vertebrae are described on the basis of the position of the articular process in the cervical region, transverse process in the thoracic region, and mammillary process in the lumbar region. The pelvic bones are listed as right or left posterior or anterior innominate bone, or right or left anterior, posterior or inferior sacrum.

Listings tell the chiropractor what his 'line of drive' should be

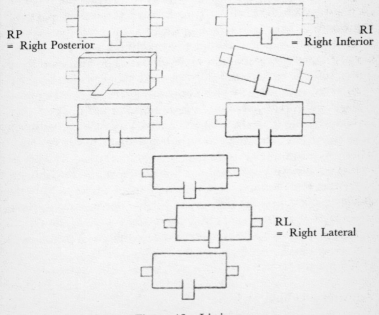

Figure 12   Listings

— that is, in which precise direction he must adjust the subluxated vertebra. Those who speak in terms of listings speak of subluxation of a vertebra. By convention, when there is a fixation, it is the upper vertebra of a pair which is considered subluxated, and the chiropractor speaks of adjusting the upper vertebra.

## Palmer Toggle Recoil Adjustment

The Palmer toggle recoil adjustment described by B. J. Palmer is used by HIO upper cervical pratitioners, who restrict their adjusting to the atlas and occasionally the axis. This adjustment can, however, be used on any vertebra and even on the pelvis. It has been briefly described in chapter 1. It is worth explaining it once more as it is, I believe, part of the reason why chiropractic is so successful. It gives the practitioner speed and precision.

The wrist of the contact hand is grasped with the other in such a way that the pisiform bone (the small round carpal bone below and in front of the base of the little finger at the wrist) is in the hollow formed at the base of the thumb when the thumb is outstretched (the anatomical snuffbox). The arms are hung down from the shoulders in such a way that one pisiform bone is directly over the other, which in turn contacts the vertebra to be moved. The chiropractor relaxes his arms totally, then suddenly straightens the elbows which act as a toggle sending a very rapid low amplitude impulse on to the contact vertebra. There is an immediate recoil action.

It is the fastest type of adjustment possible and is the ultimate rapid-thrust technique. It is through this technique that the chiropractor learns to acquire a high-velocity action. It is essential that chiropractors learn to produce a rapid impulse in adjusting. That is what characterizes the chiropractic adjustment and indeed what makes it different from other forms of manipulation.

## Adjusting Tables

To match different techniques, different tables are used by

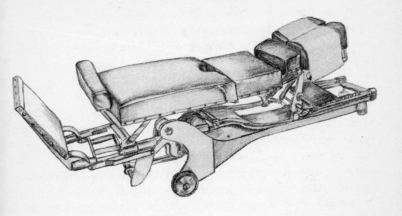

Figure 13    The Hi-Lo Chiropractic Table

chiropractors, some with variations to suit their particular methods. Since adjustments, particularly of the thoracic spine, are made with the patient face-down, a split headpiece, on which the patient can lie with his nose and mouth in the gap between two cushions, or at least a hole in the head end of the table to allow the patient to breathe, is essential. It is said that D. D. Palmer caused many a nosebleed adjusting on his table with a solid headpiece! A method of adjusting which used to be used was to have the patient kneeling with only his chest and head supported. From this was developed the adjusting table in two sections, with chest and abdominal section and thigh section which can be moved apart, and a split headpiece which can be tilted forwards. Further refinements are the facility of raising the abdominal and thigh cushions at an angle, to accommodate patients who, because of a disc lesion, may be unable to lie flat or straighten up, and a sprung abdominal section which allows the abdomen to drop when pressure is applied to the back. A motor, which enables the whole table to be raised or lowered from horizontal to an almost vertical position, is another option. The patient simply stands on a footplate and goes down with the table, his ankles being supported by another cushioned section. This motorized table is known as a Hi-lo. There are versions in which the whole table in the horizontal position can be raised and lowered to suit the height of the chiropractor, and others with swivelling sections as well.

Drop section tables have sections which can be raised before adjustment in such a way that as soon as a sudden force is applied vertically the section drops an inch or two. A separate rest for the head is obtainable which drops when a toggle adjustment is performed. The idea is that very little force is applied, as the neck immediately moves away from the adjusting hand. It also protects the adjustor's shoulders from taking the force of the adjustment. Similar drop pieces are available on some tables for any part of the body. One disadvantage of the toggle recoil adjustment is that it is usually quite silent. There is no joint crack. Both chiropractor and patient find the joint crack useful because it shows them that a joint really has been moved. The drop headpiece, or other drop section, makes a click as it drops, which makes the adjustment sound more effective.

There is no doubt that apparatus such as special tables can be very useful. It is not essential, however, and there is no need to take tables to visit patients in their own homes. Their bed, a chair, or whatever furniture is available can be used. A chiropractor's tools are his hands. He can do without machines.

## Adjustment

We have seen that there are various schools and systems of chiropractic. There are also varieties of tables to suit different methods and personal tastes. What then is it that characterizes chiropractic and makes it different from other forms of spinal manipulative therapy? It is the adjustment. Joints which have become fixed are freed by a movement which is small in amplitude, ultra-rapid, and uses little force. It is applied to one of the vertebrae adjacent to the fixation, often using one of the processes of the vertebraa as a lever. The contact point and direction are specific enough to be able to separate the articular surfaces of an individual joint.

## Chapter 8

# Dilemmas

**Risk of Chiropractic**

The safety of chiropractic manipulation has been dicussed in chapter 1. It is remarkably safe. No effective treatments are completely without risks, but these are minimized if the chiropractor is aware of factors in the patient's medical history which may be contra-indications to particular manipulations or reasons for caution. Acute injuries of the neck — for instance, those due to road accidents — should have X-ray studies to check the absence of fractures and dislocations before treatment is started. Certain diseases such as rheumatoid arthritis and ankylosing spondylitis can lead to loosening of the ligaments at the top of the neck with dislocation of the axis vertebra which can press on the spinal cord. The chiropractor should be aware of these conditions and make the appropriate X-ray studies or avoid manipulating the neck. Stroke following manipulation of the neck has been described. It is very rare but is a reason for caution in those with arteriosclerosis of the arteries of the neck.

Obviously, if the bones of the spine are crumbling — for instance, because of cancer or tuberculosis — manipulations could be dangerous. X-rays or bone scans using radioisotopes will reveal the position, and it would be ususual for a chiropractor not to realize that there was severe disease present through the tenderness elicited on palpation and the general 'feel' of the spine.

Severe prolapsed lumbar intervertebral discs can be made worse by manipulation. The technique used can be adapted to minimize this possibility. Should a manipulation appear to have aggravated a disc lesion, however, a chiropractor can often help by manipulating other areas of the spine which will have a beneficial effect on the mechanics of the spine as a whole. In cases of severe deterioration, of course, he may refer the patient for surgical treatment.

Apart from such cases where there are contra-indications or reasons for caution, chiropractic adjustments are safe and it is more likely that harm will be done by not treating. If a joint has become lastingly fixed, to leave it in this state is to permit deterioration, whereas to free it is to encourage healing to take place. Overmanipulation is not possible if the chiropractor only manipulates where there is an indication. Manipulation, even of normal joints, does not appear to cause significant harm (although such manipulation would be pointless).

### Lack of Improvement

If the patient feels no improvement after a number of treatment sessions, he should discuss his worries with his chiropractor. It may be that the chiropractor can see objective improvement which the patient cannot, and assure the patient that subjective improvement will follow. If the chiropractor feels improvement is not happening sufficiently quickly, he may wish to investigate further, perhaps with X-rays or blood tests, to review the diagnosis. He may refer the patient for further investigation, or for a different kind of treatment, usually through his general practitioner.

There can be no hard-and-fast rules about when lack of progress means seeking an alternative route. It must be a matter of agreement between the chiropractor and the patient. If the patient is not happy with his chiropractor's assessment of the situation, he should request another opinion, which should never be refused.

### Dependence

A patient may worry that treatment will weaken the spine in some way so that he has to keep being treated to stay right. He can be reassured that this is not so. The idea that chiropractic can be of temporary benefit but does not cause permanent improvement is also the opposite of the truth. There can, however, be a kind of dependence on treatment. The patient can feel insecure after a few weeks without treatment, and think things are going wrong when they are not. As in other fields, an insecure patient can develop a psychological dependence on the therapist. This situation should be recognized by the chiropractor and faced frankly, so that the patient is actively discouraged from coming more than is absolutely necessary. It should be be recognized, however, that some patients do require regular manipulations over a long period, or even indefinitely, to keep longstanding conditions under control. In other words, treatment may be directed towards maintaining the state of health (preventative rather than curative). Patients should never be afraid to ask questions, and the chiropractor should be ready to explain his diagnosis, and the aim of treatment. In this way, the chiropractor understands the patient's needs and expectations, and the patient understands what the chiropractor is able to do, and what he trying to achieve.

## Masking of Diseases

The possibility of chiropractic treatment concealing a disease, because the patient feels better, is a real one. Often patients with pain from cancers, with symptoms of neurological disease such as multiple sclerosis or brain tumours, or other diseases, feel better and have a reduction of symptoms after chiropractic treatment. They can then be falsely reassured that they are improving and delay receiving the correct treatment. This of course applies with other therapies. Giving anti-inflammatory or painkilling drugs can do the same. It is vital that patients are properly examined and necessary investigations carried out so that their diseases are not mis-diagnosed and mis-managed. For this reason the greater co-operation between chiropractors and doctors of recent years is welcomed. Openness on the part of the patient about who is treating what, and communication between all those treating him, are an essential to good management. With such co-operation, failing to diagnose underlying disease should be extremely uncommon. Chiropractors are thoroughly trained to recognize conditions which should be passed to another specialist. The general practitioner remains the key figure in communication. The more aware are general practitioners of the contribution chiropractic can make to the welfare of their patients, the greater will be the progress in the treatment of back pain and other distressing complaints, and the collaboration between chiropractors and other disciplines in the overall care of patients.

# Chapter 9

# The Future

In Great Britain, the general practitioner is firmly established as the doctor of primary contact for health care, and the co-ordinator of health services for his patient. There seems little point in chiropractors attempting to usurp that role. On the other hand, even if spinal manipulative therapy does become part of the general practitioners' training, they will not be able to devote sufficient time to training or to the practice of this work. Physiotherapy is expanding with new modalities and new methods of re-education and rehabilitation, and has an increasingly important part to play in the care of hospital inpatients as well as in the community. But neither physiotherapists nor general practitioners can take over the function of chiropractors in spinal manipulative therapy.

The future lies in communication, co-operation and teamwork. The work of the chiropractor and the physiotherapist are complementary. The work of general practitioners, orthopaedic surgeons, rheumatologists, neurologists and neurosurgeons and chiropractors are also complementary. They will need increasingly to work together to treat and control back pain and musculoskeletal disorders.

The other and larger group of manipulative practitioners in Britain are the osteopaths. Perhaps, in time, the various groups of osteopaths will come together and osteopaths and chiropractors will learn to pool their resources, and maybe even become one profession. It seems unlikely that either group will become recognized and officially registered by the State while excluding the other.

The British Chiropractic Association trial of chiropractic versus hospital outpatient treatment for back pain which is now under way, heralds an era not only for necessary research to prove the efficacy of chiropractic treatment, but also of equally necessary co-operation between chiropractors and medical practitioners. After ninety-one years of chiropractic, things are only just beginning to move, but the future looks bright. We have a strong and united chiropractic profession in Great Britain. We have a chiropractic college. Acceptance of the excellent course at the Anglo-European College of Chiropractic as a bachelor's degree course seems likely to happen fairly soon. Recognition and registration of the profession, leading to chiropractic being included as a normal part of health care in the National Health Service would seem to be very much in the interest of our society and may not be too far off.

In spite of opposition from very powerful groups in the USA, chiropractic refused to die and has grown to maturity. In Great Britain, it is still in its infancy, but it is growing and increasing in strength of numbers, in wisdom, in knowledge and in achievement.

# Useful Addresses

## Great Britain

Anglo-European College of Chiropractic
Arne Christensen, DC, Dean
13–15 Parkwood Road
Boscombe
Bournemouth
Dorset BH5 2DF
Tel: 0202 431021

British Chiropractic Association
Susan L. Moore, DC
Executive Secretary
Ground Floor
1 Arthington Avenue
Harrogate
N. Yorkshire HG1 5NB
Tel: 0423 525863

The Chiropractic Advancement Association
Mrs Betty Kenny, Secretary
38a Upper Richmond Road West
London SW14
Tel: 01–878–3989

## Europe

The European Chiropractors' Union
A. M. Metcalfe, DC, Hon. Secretary
19 Strawberry Hill Road
Twickenham
Middlesex, Great Britain
Tel: 01 892 3940

## North America

American Chiropractic Association
G. M. Brassard, DC, Executive Vice President
1916 Wilson Blvd.
Arlington
Virginia 22201 USA

Canadian Chiropractic Association
J. L. Watkins, DC, Executive Vice President
290, Lawrence Avenue West
Toronto
Ontario, M5M 1B3 Canada

International Chiropractors Association
Bruce E. Nordstrom, DC, Executive Vice President
1901 L Street, N.W. Suite 800
Washington DC 20036 USA

# Index